Experimental Embryology
of Echinoderms

Sven Hörstadius

Experimental Embryology
of Echinoderms

CLARENDON PRESS · OXFORD
1973

Oxford University Press, Ely House, London W. 1

GLASGOW   NEW YORK   TORONTO   MELBOURNE   WELLINGTON
CAPE TOWN   IBADAN   NAIROBI   DAR ES SALAAM   LUSAKA   ADDIS ABABA
DELHI   BOMBAY   CALCUTTA   MADRAS   KARACHI   LAHORE   DACCA
KUALA LUMPUR   SINGAPORE   HONG KONG   TOKYO

PRINTED IN GREAT BRITAIN
BY THE PITMAN PRESS, BATH

Preface

THIS book would probably never have been written but for the encouragement offered, more than ten years ago, by my old friend the late Sir Gavin de Beer. It was he who suggested, and then made me promise to write, a book with the title *Experimental Embryology of Echinoderms*.

The book is addressed principally to two groups of people. The one group comprises young students of zoology, particularly those who intend to take up research; my hope is to introduce them to a fascinating field. The other group includes all scientists using embryological echinoderm material in their studies. Too often researchers in cytology, physiology, and molecular biology have little or no knowledge of the morphogenetic properties of their material and lack appreciation of the long and enthralling process by which such knowledge has been obtained. As a historical perspective is interesting and, indeed, essential for understanding the problems, I have endeavoured, however briefly, to give due credit to the pioneers.

I am deeply grateful to Professor Tryggve Gustafson and Dr. Berndt Hagström, both of Stockholm, who have read the typescript and given much good advice. My sincere thanks are due also to Professor George Hughes of Bristol who, on receiving from me the first chapters with a request that he seek a young zoologist willing to correct my English, preferred to undertake that heavy task himself. The major part of the typescript, however, has been corrected by Mr. F. P. Walsh, Stockholm. The final trimming I owe to the painstaking efforts of the Clarendon Press. Mrs. Kerstin Ahlfors and Mrs. Nanna Gustafsson of the technical staff of the Zoological Institute, Uppsala, have with great skill assisted in preparing the illustrations.

Uppsala, November 1972   S. H.

Acknowledgements

The illustrations are reproduced by courtesy of the following publishers and journals: Academic Press (*Chemical Zoology, Developmental Biology, Experimental Cell Research*); *Acta Embryologiae Experimentalis; Acta Zoologica*, Stockholm; Akademische Verlagsgesellschaft (*Zeitschrift für wissenschaftliche Zoologie*); *American Scientist; L'Année Biologique*; Birkhäuser Verlag (F. E. Lehmann: *Einführung in die physiologische Embryologie*); Cambridge University Press (*Biological Reviews*); The Company of Biologists Ltd. (*Journal of Embryology and Experimental Morphology*); Gustav Fischer Verlag, Jena (*Anatomischer Anzeiger; Zoologische Jahrbücher, Abt. Anatomie und Ontogenie*); Gustav Fischer Verlag, Stuttgart (*Jena Zeitschrift für Naturwissenschaften*); Institut Royal des Sciences Naturelles de Belgique (*Mémoires de Musée Royal d'Histoire Naturelle*); Kungl. Vetenskapsakademien (*Arkiv för Zoologi*); *Pubblicazione della Stazione Zoologica di Napoli*; The Royal Society of London (*Philosophical Transactions*); Springer Verlag (*Die Naturwissenschaften. A. Kühn: Vorlesungen über die Entwicklungsphysiologie*); Urban und Schwarzenberg (*Abderhaldens Handbuch der biologischen Arbeitsmethoden*); Verlag J. F. Bergmann (*Wilhelm Roux' Archiv für Entwicklungsmechanik der Organismen*); Verlag der *Zeitschrift für Naturforschung;* The Wistar Institute Press (*Journal of Experimental Zoology*).

Contents

1 *Introduction*

A professor of zoology started to tell his six-year-old son how animals come into existence from a small egg. He showed him drawings in a textbook of how an egg divides into many cells, and told him that there would be an enormous number of them, and that eventually they would form the different tissues and organs of the body. With the clear logic of a child the boy asked: 'But, Daddy, how do the cells know which of them are going to form those organs?' Yes, how do they know? That, in a nutshell, is the problem of experimental embryology and developmental physiology.

Cleavage cells as a rule resemble each other, are spherical, and as yet unadapted for their future life as part of organs. Differentiation implies their transformation into cells of special shape and structure, capable of certain functions, and forming characteristic tissues. Movements of cell layers and the appearance of different tissues create the shape of the larvae: morphogenesis. Early cleavage cells often have capacity to differentiate in another way than they normally should have done. If they have been isolated or brought into contact with cells other than their normal neighbours or affected by chemicals they may participate in the formation of tissues and organs of quite another kind from those corresponding to their normal development. However, in the course of development the potencies of cells become restricted to a given pathway; the cell can then only differentiate in one direction. To analyse this process, generally called determination, is the major objective of this book.

An early experiment (see Fig. 12) proved that differentiation is not due to a distribution of qualitatively different nuclei. The genomes reaching different parts of the body are alike; the differentiation of each cell depends on an interaction between nucleus and adjacent cytoplasm.

The properties of the cytoplasm of different regions of the egg are therefore of paramount importance, directing the way of differentiation. The pathway of the cell is not, however, irrevocably specified solely by the relationship between nucleus and cytoplasm; it is also to a great extent dependent on environmental influence—first, through internal factors such as interactions with surrounding cells and secondly through external factors such as temperature or chemicals.

This book is not concerned with growth *sensu stricto*, that is, increase of total mass by incorporation from the exterior. Real growth allowing further diversification of shape and organs starts after assimilation of food; another example is the enlargement of the oocyte by absorption of substances brought by neighbouring cells. The increase in volume of a larva because of formation of thin epithelia as well as, for example, the first elongation of arms and skeletal rods of early larvae, are only consequences of differentiation and do not justly earn the designation growth.

One of the most important objects of studies in experimental biology has been the sea-urchin egg. There are several reasons for this: (a) artificial fertilization is readily achieved and hence desired stages of development can be obtained at any time; (b) the larvae are transparent, as are also the eggs of some species, and thus allow microscopical studies of the living material to be made; (c) eggs can be obtained in large quantities, which facilitates physiological and biochemical investigations; (d) the regular type of cleavage makes possible work with fragments of known size and origin; (e) the egg axis is recognizable by the characteristic 16-cell stage and in one species (*Paracentrotus lividus*) the axis is already visible in the mature egg because of a pigment ring below the equator; (f) furthermore, ripe ova and sperm are available for long periods from several species, so that by choosing suitable marine stations it is possible to work on the development of sea-urchins at all times of the year.

The scope of this book is chiefly the review of the experimental results obtained by mechanical means. For this reason the old name experimental embryology is suitable. It has also been necessary to deal with some physiological problems and processes, thus entering into the wider field of developmental physiology, and even to trespass on genetics, which is included within the still wider concept of developmental biology. However, these digressions as a rule also make use of mechanical methods. An adequate presentation of investigations concerning metabolism during the course of development and its effect on determination would require another book. The main intention has not been to give as concise an account as possible of the present state of our knowledge in these fields, but rather to give credit to the many early investigations in order to show how problems have been posed and attacked with gradually more refined methods.

2 The birth and early development of experimental embryology

GREAT attention was attracted by the statement of a young German doctor, Wilhelm Roux, at a congress in Wiesbaden in 1887 that a half tadpole-larva had developed from one of the first two blastomeres of a frog egg after the other cell had been killed with a hot needle. The results were published (1888a) under the title 'Ueber die künstliche Hervorrufung halber Embryonen nach Zerstörung einer der beiden ersten Furchungskugeln, sowie über die Nachentwickelung (Postgeneration) der fehlenden Körperhälfte'. This paper has been called a milestone in biology. Roux had obtained left and right halves with only one row of somites, and later with only a lateral half of the neural plate. He drew the conclusion that the first cleavage furrow had divided the presumptive left and right halves from each other. In other cases he found anterior half-embryos with only the head part of the neural plate, and gave the explanation that in these eggs not the first, but the second furrow had coincided with the median plane. The results led Roux to the conception that different parts of the egg are qualitatively different and that the cells in early stages are determined to form specific parts of the body, constituting a mosaic of independently differentiating pieces. Roux speaks of a 'self-differentiation' of the blastomeres, implying that they contain not only the material but also the necessary forces for differentiating the material of the fragment in the same way as would have occurred in the whole larva.

When Roux further observed that the half-embryos soon began to be transformed into complete larvae of half-size, he called this process 'postgeneration'. The word 'generation' could not be used as the missing parts had not existed before. Roux explained this phenomenon by the assumption that only activated material is qualitatively separated at cleavage and that material also exists in an inactive state which can be set working under abnormal conditions. Thanks to the studies of Hans Spemann we now know that the first two blastomeres of amphibian eggs when separated from each other will provide complete dwarf larvae, given that they represent lateral or dorsal halves; whereas ventral halves do not develop chorda and neural tissue because of the absence of the organizing region of the dorsal lip of the blastopore.

Roux, however, was not the first to present results of this kind. The previous year Chabry (1887) killed one of the first two blastomeres of ascidian eggs and observed mosaic cleavage and differentiation, but this paper did not attract the same attention. It is possible that the work was indirectly based on Roux's first paper in the series, 'Beiträge zur Entwickelungsmechanik des Embryo' (1885), in which he described the use of hot steel needles, and which he had sent to Chabry's teacher G. Pouchet. There are two reasons for particularly mentioning Chabry's paper here: he invented an apparatus for the operations employing very fine glass needles, forerunners of the tools of Spemann which have played such a decisive role in experimental embryology; and secondly, Chabry presents two drawings of an egg of *Paracentrotus lividus*, the first showing the egg pierced right through by a glass needle, and the second showing the needle withdrawn leaving an internal scar. Nevertheless this egg developed into a pluteus, a first example of the ability of sea-urchin eggs to endure rough treatment by experimenters. Roux himself called the new experimental branch of embryology 'Entwickelungsmechanik' (mechanics of development), but the name developmental physiology is now generally accepted, a designation covering not only experiments with operative methods but also studies of metabolic processes of significance for determination and differentiation.

Within a few years the early results and interpretations of Roux were contradicted by experiments on the eggs of echinoderms. Oscar and Richard Hertwig (1887) found that shaking could fragment such eggs into pieces with or without nuclei. Both kinds of fragments could be fertilized and start cleavage. Two years later Theodor Boveri stated that fragments of sea-urchin eggs after fertilization could develop further and form small plutei, a proof that an egg can develop to a larva although deprived of part of its material. It was another young German, Hans Driesch, who more systematically tried to analyse the qualities of different areas of sea-urchin eggs by studying the development of fragments. In his first experiments Driesch (1891, 1892) used the shaking method of the Hertwigs. In the following years (1892, 1893a) he applied higher temperature (31 °C) or diluted sea-water to facilitate the separation of blastomeres. Considerable progress was made when Curt Herbst (1900) found that cleavage cells fall apart when brought into artificial sea-water without calcium ions. By pre-treatment with calcium-free sea-water and only slight shaking Driesch obtained a variety of fragments composed of different numbers and types of cleavage cells. He found that isolated blastomeres of the 2- and 4-cell stages segmented in the same way as would have occurred in the whole egg (Fig. 1(a)), but in spite of the half- or quarter-cleavage they could develop into small plutei (Fig. 1(b)–(d)). These results tallied with those of Roux with respect

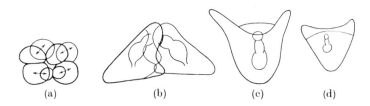

FIG. 1. (a) Half-cleavage of half-blastomere. (b) Partly fused twin plutei from the two half-blastomeres of one egg. (c, d) Plutei from isolated half- and quarter-blastomeres. (a, b) *Psammechinus microtuberculatus*, (c, d) *Sphaerechinus granularis*. (From Driesch 1891, 1900*a*.)

to the mosaic type of cleavage, but the discovery that fragments developed into whole larvae was sensational and opened a new line of research.

Fragments of 8-cell stages did not give such uniform results. Isolation in this stage is important as the third, equatorial, furrow separates the animal, purely ectodermal, half from the vegetal half containing the future endoderm and mesoderm material. In the 16-cell stage the animal half consists of 8 cells of medium size, the mesomeres, and the vegetal half of 4 large macromeres and 4 small micromeres. Driesch judged fragments forming macro- and micromeres to be meridional or vegetal, and those with cells of equal size to be animal; he found that some of the latter type could give plutei while others remained as blastulae with enlarged animal tuft. In spite of these exceptions he considered the sea-urchin egg as a 'harmonious equipotential system'.

On these results Driesch built his vitalistic philosophy, speaking of the 'autonomy of life processes', the importance of 'das Ganze' (the whole), and presuming a certain non-physical force, the 'entelechy', necessary to explain the power of regulation (1901). He persisted with this doctrine in spite of other work contradicting the interpretation of the sea-urchin egg as an harmonious equipotential system. Zoja (1895), Boveri (1901*b*, 1902), and Terni (1914) stated that animal halves never gastrulate. In his classic paper Boveri 1901*b* advanced the hypothesis of a stratification along the animal–vegetal axis of the sea-urchin egg, and he also used the word 'Gefälle' (gradient) in this connexion (1901*b*, 1910*a*). Instead of relying on a mysterious force, regulation could be considered as depending on the constitution of the egg. The main arguments of Driesch had collapsed as they were based on erroneous observations and an experimental error (see pages 19–22 and 42).

As Driesch had made the remarkable discovery that, according to its circumstances, a part of an egg can give rise to other parts of the larva than it would have formed in normal development, he introduced the terms 'prospektive Bedeutung' (prospective significance) and 'prospektive Potenz' (prospective potency). The former term indicates the actual fate of the material in normal development, while the latter signifies all the developmental possibilities of a part of the egg. The term 'totipotency' is used when a fragment has the capacity to form all kinds of tissues and organs of a larva. 'Pluripotency' means the faculty for more diversified differentiation than corresponds to prospective significance, short of totipotency. The word 'presumptive' is often used to denote the prospective significance of a part, for example, presumptive endoderm.

As mentioned above, Roux used the word self-differentiation to denote a differentiation of a fragment in accordance with the prospective significance of the material. However, the word is ambiguous. Every fragment capable of development differentiates by itself. Real self-differentiation in the sense meant by Roux is relatively rare. The word has sometimes been used to describe the development of fragments independently of the way the differentiation takes place, even when it leads to a typical larva of reduced size or produces something differing both from a dwarf and a mosaic piece. To avoid misunderstanding it is therefore preferable to speak of the result of the development of all fragments as their autonomous differentiation, whatever line it may follow, while reserving the term self-differentiation for only one of them, strictly in accordance with the prospective significance of the material (Hörstadius 1938, p. 240).

The discoveries made on eggs of amphibians and sea-urchins gave impetus to investigations of the same kind in other groups. Similar results, with a certain amount of regulation, were found in *Amphioxus* and nemertines (Wilson 1892*a*, 1903), in the fish *Fundulus* (Morgan 1893,

1895*f*), in Hydrozoa (Zoja 1895; Maas 1901, 1905), and in cyclostomes (Bataillon 1900). In contrast to these results were observations on eggs of which fragments developed as they normally should have done—that is, the egg consisting of a mosaic of self-differentiating regions (ascidians, Chabry 1887; Conklin 1905*a, b,* 1906: ctenophores, Chun 1892; Driesch and Morgan 1895: *Nereis* and *Patella*, Wilson 1896, 1904). In the course of these investigations some evidence of progressive changes as well as of interactions between parts of the egg were demonstrated. Roux (1888*b*) was the first to observe the formation of the grey crescent after fertilization of the amphibian egg. In the egg of *Myzostoma*, Driesch (1896*b*) and Wheeler (1898) saw a remodelling of cytoplasms of different character at fertilization and maturation. Conklin (1905*a, b*) described cytoplasmic movements in the fertilized ascidian egg leading to a specific distribution of substances of different appearance and with different tasks. The fact that removal of one part of the egg could lead to defects, even lack of an organ in another part (*Dentalium*, Wilson 1904) led to the opinion that 'organ-forming substances' may act at a distance. In the early days it was generally believed that there was a significant difference between regulation and mosaic eggs. Later investigations have shown, however, that the latter are not always so strictly mosaic. There are only differences in the time when cells lose the faculty of regulation and become strictly determined.

Basic contributions to genetics were made by Boveri (1902, 1908) in his studies of eggs fertilized with more than one sperm (polyspermy). If two sperms penetrate into an egg the result may be formation of three or four spindles and abnormal distribution of the chromosomes, leading to defects in different parts of the body (see Fig. 70). From such observations Boveri was able to prove not only that chromosomes are carriers of heredity but also that they are qualitatively different (see Chapter 9).

Curt Herbst was a pioneer in the field of developmental physiology. He stated in a number of papers (1892–1906) that changes in the composition of the sea-water, and particularly the addition of some substances to it, influence differentiation and may lead, for example, to an increase of endoderm at the expense of presumptive ectoderm or, vice versa, strengthening of the ectodermal properties. An important step for the advancement of physiological studies was the measurement by Otto Warburg (1908) of respiration in unfertilized eggs and developing larvae. Fertilization caused an immediate six- to seven-fold increase in oxygen consumption, followed by a slow increase during early development.

Although in 1906 Spemann had recommended fine glass needles for operations on sea-urchins they were not used on echinoderms until two decades later (von Ubisch 1925*b*; Hörstadius 1925*b*). Vogt's method of local vital staining with small pieces of agar (1925) was also first applied to sea-urchins by von Ubisch (1925*a*). With these two methods new ways were opened for a more accurate analysis of the morphological events and interactions between different regions during the development of sea-urchin eggs and larvae.

3 *Normal early development of sea-urchin larvae*

A prerequisite for experimental work is a thorough knowledge of the normal development.

The first report of artificial insemination and of development to pluteus stage was published by Derbès 1847 (*Echinus esculentus*). The same year also von Baer described cleavage and development to swimming blastula of the same species. Fol (1877, 1879) was the first to observe the penetration of a sperm through jelly layer and entrance cone (cône d'attraction) into eggs of the starfish *Asterias glacialis* and the sea-urchin *Paracentrotus lividus*. Shortly before, Oscar Hertwig (1876), with stained sections of eggs of the same sea-urchin species, had been able to demonstrate the true significance of fertilization—fusion of egg and sperm nuclei. Other early studies of sea-urchin development we owe to Selenka (1878, 1883).

The egg axis is often called the animal–vegetal axis. These terms were probably used for the first time by von Baer (1828) with respect to the germ layers of the chick. Animal cells give rise to ectoderm which differentiates not only to skin but also to neural system which is an innovation of animals. Vegetal cells are the source of the greater part of the digestive tract upon which the further growth of the larva depends.

The sea-urchin egg

In the ovary the young oocytes are attached to the wall by a broad base. The oocyte gradually rounds up and the connexion with the wall is transformed to a narrow stem. The oocyte is only partly covered by thin follicle cells. It appears that the nutriment for growth is brought to the oocyte more by migratory cells than through the adjacent epithelial cells or the follicle. The oocyte is surrounded by a jelly layer which in sea-water will swell considerably to a thickness of about 20 μm (Fig. 2). The jelly coat cannot be seen in sea-water but becomes visible in coloured water, in water with suspended small particles, or if it is stained. At the pole opposite the stem a plug penetrates the jelly layer, thereby forming the micropyle canal. Here the polar bodies are budded off (Fig. 2(b), (c)). The egg axis, with the animal pole at the free micropyle end, is evidently determined already when the growing oocyte is fixed to the ovarian wall. (Boveri 1901*a*; Jenkinson 1911*b*; Lindahl 1932*a*, 1941*a*).

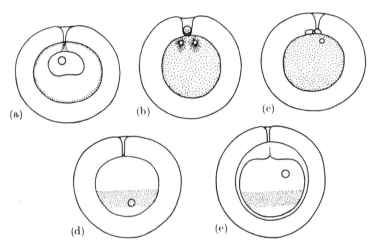

FIG. 2. (a) Oocyte of *Paracentrotus lividus* with germinal vesicle with nucleolus, micropyle through the jelly coat. (b), (c) Maturation process, formation of the polar bodies: pigment granules still evenly distributed. (d) Mature egg, pigment concentrated to a band below the equator. (e) Fertilized egg with raised fertilization membrane. (Redrawn from Boveri 1901*a*.)

A single sea-urchin egg may be difficult to detect with the naked eye as the diameter is often less than a tenth of a millimetre. Lönning and Wennerberg (1963) have given mean values from three European stations, Naples(N), Espegrend in Norway(E), and Kristineberg in Sweden(K). The shortest diameter was found for *Arbacia lixula* (N) with 79·3 μm. This should be compared with the rather similar figure (74 μm) for the American *A. punctulata* (Harvey 1956). The next smaller eggs were *Paracentrotus lividus* (N) (93·2 μm) and *Psammechinus miliaris* (K) (96·6 μm). At Kristineberg the salinity is considerably lower than in the ocean. The eggs of the same species on the Atlantic coast of Norway (E) measured 115·0 μm. The eggs of *Psammechinus micro-tuberculatus* (N), *Sphaerechinus granularis* (N) and *Brissopsis lyrifera* (K) are of moderate size (about 100 μm), while *Echinus esculentus* (E) and *Strongylocentrotus droebachiensis* (E) are 'giants', with eggs of 153·4 and 145·6 μm respectively.

There is no easily visible stratification of yolk or other substances in the interior of the eggs. The *Arbacia* egg is strongly pigmented. Morgan (1894) observed that the pigment at the 4-cell stage moves away from the pole where the micromeres will be formed. Of particular interest and importance is the type of pigmentation found in the eggs of *Paracentrotus lividus*. The surface of the oocyte is covered with a faintly reddish, evenly distributed pigment (Fig. 2(a)–(c)). At maturation the pigment migrates from the animal half and from the vegetal pole to form a girdle below the equator (d) (Selenka 1883; Boveri 1901a). This pigment band is not clearly seen in the eggs of many batches but when well developed it indicates the polarity clearly enough for experimental purposes. The band is said to be better developed in eggs from Villefranche than in those from Naples. A few cases with the pigment ring in an oblique position with respect to the egg axis have been reported (Selenka 1883; Garbowski 1905), but they occur very rarely, perhaps never in healthy eggs. Such an event can practically be ignored in experimental work: probably in some cases the ring did not stand obliquely in relation to the egg axis, but did so to an oblique cleavage axis (Hörstadius 1928). In other species the polarity can be traced only by the location of the polar bodies and the micropyle.

Fertilization, a much debated process

In some marine animals the maturation of oocytes starts only after contact with sea-water or after fertilization. In the sea-urchin this process is already complete in the ovary before natural spawning. The unfertilized egg represents a resting stage. Fertilization has a twofold effect. The first is incorporation of the sperm into the egg with eventual fusion of egg and sperm nuclei. The second is activation of the egg involving onset of mitotic activity and increase of metabolism, for example, the transient production of a strong acid (Runnström 1933), the rise of respiration (Warburg 1908), the increase of protein and nucleic acid synthesis and enzymatic activities.

An extensive literature exists on the different aspects of fertilization. In this book it is possible to mention only briefly the main results and problems. For reviews of this vast field see, for instance, Ebert and Sussex (1970), Gustafson (1969), Monroy (1965), Rothschild (1956), Runnström (1966a), Tyler and Tyler (1966).

The long filament projecting through the jelly coat after fertilization of the *Asterias* egg was discovered by Fol (1877) who, as well as other investigators, interpreted it as an entrance cone from the egg surface. Its main part consists, however, of the everted acrosome of the sperm (Popa 1927; Dan 1956). The filament of double origin is long in starfish and holothurians but, as observed in electron micrographs, rather short in sea-urchins. The first sign of fertilization at low magnification is the elevation of the fertilization membrane (Fig. 2(e)). Elevation starts at the point of entry of the sperm a few seconds later. Full elevation is attained within about a minute, the time depending on temperature and physiological condition of the egg. The formation of the membrane is a complex process. The superficial layer of the cortex of the unfertilized egg is called the vitelline membrane, followed underneath by an equally thin so-called plasma membrane. In the cytoplasm beneath these membranes there is a layer containing cortical granules, or rather vesicles. A wave of cortical changes spreads from the point of sperm entry (Just 1919; Runnström 1923). The cortical vesicles break down or explode, their content partly fusing with the vitelline membrane to form the fertilization membrane, partly joining the plasma membrane to build up the new egg surface, the hyaline layer, which is strong enough to hold together the blastomeres during cleavage and also to allow further development in the absence of a fertilization membrane (Harvey 1910; Moser 1939; Motomura 1941; Endo 1952, 1961). In the starfish *Astropecten aranciacus* a thick preformed membrane was described and thought to be elevated without change (Hörstadius 1939b, Fig. 1). In *Asterias forbesii* the oocytes also have a thick discrete membrane. However, in electron micrographs Millonig (in Monroy 1965) found that cortical granules explode at the elevation and that part of their content joins the inside of the membrane.

The space between the fertilization membrane and the egg surface is called the perivitelline space. Osmosis seems to be involved in the elevation and expansion of the membrane (Loeb 1908; Hiramoto 1955b). From the fact that the egg occupies a central position within the membrane—not sinking under the influence of gravity—it has been concluded that the perivitelline liquid is of a jelly-like consistency (Fol 1879; Hiramoto 1954, 1955a).

Although the egg is attacked by a swarm of spermatozoa, polyspermy occurs very infrequently; the block to entrance of additional sperm must set in rather quickly. The formation of the fertilization membrane is too slow a process to seal off the egg against supernumerary sperm. It has been estimated that about 90 per cent of these are mechanically trapped or lose their fertilizing capacity during attempts to penetrate the jelly coat (Hagström 1956a,b,c, 1959). As disturbances of the cortical reactions, and consequently of the formation of the hyaline layer, lead to polyspermy, the permanent block to polyspermy has been shown to reside in the developing hyaline layer, but this localization of the process does not explain how the block really works. For surveys of recent investigations on polyspermy see Ginsburg (1968) and Lönning (1968). Activation of the egg must take place by way of the cortical layers: no activation is caused by spermatozoa injected into the cytoplasm (Chambers 1921; Hiramoto 1962), nor when they enter through a considerably damaged cortex (Runnström and Kriszat 1952a).

Frank Lillie (1912, 1919) detected in suspensions of unfertilized sea-urchin eggs a substance which agglutinates homologous sperm. This substance, which he designated fertilizin, is a component both of the jelly coat and the plasma membrane (Tyler 1948) as well as of the cortical vesicles (Motomura 1953, 1960). On the surface of sperm Lillie found a substance, antifertilizin, which at fertilization combines with fertilizin. A great number of studies have indicated that these two substances are the receptors responsible for attachment of sperm to egg. It still seems to be an open question whether chemotaxis is involved. Lillie also suggested that these substances provide the mechanism against cross fertilization between gametes from different species, thus explaining the species specificity of the gametes as a parallel to the antigen–antibody relationship.

It should be added that there is little general agreement about the interpretation of many of the aspects of fertilization.

From egg to pluteus

The spindles of the two first cleavages lie in the equatorial plane. Consequently the blastomeres of the 2- and 4-cell stages are separated by meridional furrows (see Fig. 10(a)$_2$–(a)$_4$, and Selenka 1883). These cells are of equal size. In preparing the third division the spindles have changed orientation, now parallel to the animal–vegetal axis (a)$_4$. The result is an 8-cell stage of four animal and four vegetal blastomeres (a)$_5$. As a rule the separating furrows are equatorial, again resulting in cells of equal size, but in some batches the furrows are found below the equator, the animal quartet being somewhat larger than the vegetal. Such eggs have been called subequatorial (Hörstadius 1935). The fourth cleavage produces the famous 16-cell stage (a)$_6$. The spindles in the animal quartet have changed orientation to a plane parallel to the equatorial $(a)_5$. The division leads to a ring of 8 blastomeres of equal size, the mesomeres. In the vegetal half the spindles retain the animal–vegetal direction but the cleavage is strictly unequal, giving 4 large macromeres below the equator and 4 small micromeres at the vegetal pole (Fig. $10(a)_6$, Fig. 3(d)). Before the next division the spindles have changed orientation again. The 32-cell stage (Fig. 3(e)) consists of two rings, each of 8 cells, which are designated an_1 and an_2 whereas the descendants of the macromeres have formed one ring of 8 equally sized blastomeres. The micromeres bud off 4 small micromeres. This cleavage is somewhat delayed, so that for some minutes the number of blastomeres is only 28 (Theel 1892; Zeuthen 1951; Agrell 1956a; Hagström and Lönning 1965). In the 64 cell stage (Fig. 3 (f)) the animal cells are less regularly arranged. The macromeres have now given two tiers of eight cells, each of which we call veg_1 and veg_2. The egg may thus be divided into five layers: an_1, an_2, veg_1, veg_2, and the micromeres (Hörstadius 1935).

To express the constitution of a larva from which material has been removed we shall use formulae which refer to the normal 16-cell stage: $8+4+4$ (8 mesomeres, 4 macromeres, 4 micromeres). Thus a larva from which the an_1-ring has been removed is characterized as an_2+4+4, a larva $8+veg_1+0$ is devoid of both the veg_2-ring and the micromeres, and so on.

The cell membranes become partially dissolved between micromeres, and between macro- and micromeres. Also, micromeres implanted on meso- or macromeres were found to coalesce with these latter cells in the course of a few minutes. The syncytial communication opened in this way between the micromeres and the other blastomeres may be of great importance for transport of induction agents (Hagström and Lönning 1969; Lönning and Hagström 1971).

Already during the early stages of cleavage a central cavity is formed which precedes the blastocoele. A number of cleavages with tangential spindles and radial furrows lead to the formation of a single-layered blastula wall. The mechanism has been attributed to adherence of the cells to the hyaline membrane, and changes in mechanical properties of the cell membranes (Dan 1960; Gustafson 1963). There is only a slight increase in volume during blastulation. The blastocoele contains colloid substances. Cilia appear only on the outer surface, the nuclei lying at the end towards the blastocoele. Thus a radial polarity exists. The blastula already begins rotating within the fertilization membrane;

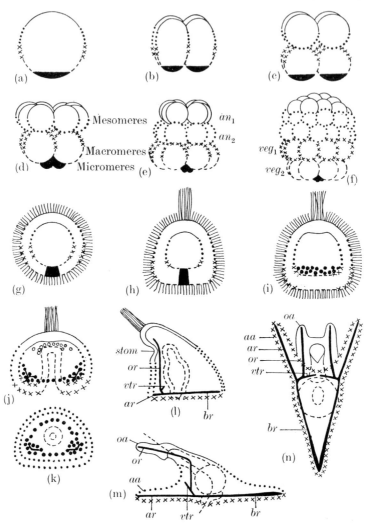

FIG. 3. Diagram of the normal development of *Paracentrotus*. Indication of the layers: an_1, continuous lines; an_2, dotted; veg_1, crosses; veg_2 broken lines; micromeres black. (a), uncleaved egg. (b), 4-cell stage. (c), 8-cell stage. (d), 16-cell stage. (e), 32-cell stage. (f), 64-cell stage. (g), young blastula. (h), later blastula, with animal tuft, before the formation of the primary mesenchyme. (i), blastula with primary mesenchyme. (j), gastrula; secondary mesenchyme and the two triradiate spicules formed. (k), transverse optical section of the same gastrula; bilateral symmetry established. (l), the so-called prism stage; stomodaeum invaginating. (m), pluteus larva from the left side; the broken line indicates the position of the egg axis. (n), pluteus from the anal side. *aa*, anal arm; *ar*, anal rod; *br*, body-rod; *oa*, oral arm; *or*, oral rod; *stom*, stomodaeum; *vtr*, ventral transverse rod. (From Hörstadius 1935, 1939a.)

when this becomes dissolved by a hatching enzyme the blastula starts swimming in spiral courses towards the surface. At the animal pole the active cilia are replaced by a tuft of long, immovable cilia, stereocilia. They remain throughout the blastula and gastrula to the prism stage (Fig. 3(h)–(l)). The function of this organ is probably to detect contact with the surface layer of the water. A young larva caught by the surface film is disrupted by the tension, the soft cell layer being spread out. The contact of the tuft with the film may lead to a change in the direction of swimming. The tuft is usually called the apical or ciliary tuft. As the most dorsal point of the pluteus larva is known as the apex (see Fig. 5) the word apical is rather misleading. We prefer to call this organ the animal tuft.

Already before gastrulation cells from the vegetal pole migrate into the blastocoele as primary mesenchyme cells which later give rise to the skeleton (Fig. 3(i), Fig. 4(a), (b)). Boveri (1901*a*, *b*) observed that these cells are derived from the unpigmented vegetal cap which forms the micromeres during cleavage. This observation was confirmed by isolation, vital staining and replacement of micromeres (Hörstadius 1935, p. 279).

The old blastula is no longer a sphere. The vegetal side is flattened and thicker than the meridional sides. The region of the animal tuft also has a higher epithelium (Fig. 3(i)). The vegetal wall keeps its shape also after immigration of the primary mesenchyme. From this plate the archenteron is invaginated (Fig. 3(i), (j), Fig. 4(c), (d), Fig. 6). At the tip of the archenteron the secondary mesenchyme and the coelom are budded off (Fig. 3(j), Fig. 4(e)). At this stage we find the first traces of bilateral symmetry. One side of the gastrula is flattened and remains thicker than the other sides (Fig. 3(k), Fig. 4(d–f)), developing into the oral field surrounded by the ciliated band, the most animal part of which corresponds to the plate with the animal tuft, the animal plate or acron (Fig. 3(l), Fig. 4(e), (f), Fig. 5). The primary mesenchyme cells in the ring round the base of the archenteron concentrate more at the corners of the ventral side and secrete two triradiate spicules, the beginning of the skeleton (Fig. 3(j), (k), Fig. 4(e)).

The archenteron is divided into oesophagus, stomach, and intestine. The oesophagus is bent towards the ventral side where it will meet and fuse with an ectodermal ingrowth, the stomodaeum (Fig. 3(l), (m), Fig. 4(f), (h), Fig. 5). Therefore the mouth and the oral cavity are of ectodermal origin. Some of the secondary mesenchyme cells form the muscular bands of the alimentary canal (Fig. 4(h)). Others contain granules of red

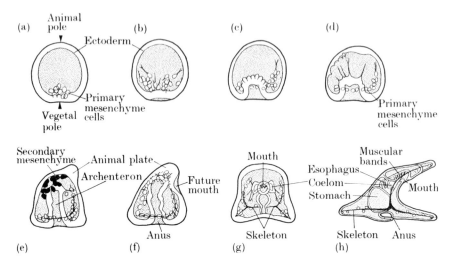

FIG. 4. Some stages in the early development of *Psammechinus miliaris*.
(a), (b) Primary mesenchyme cells released from the vegetal blastula wall.
(c) First step of invagination of the archenteron. (d) Beginning of the
second step with exploring pseudopods from the cells of the tip of the
archenteron. (e), (f) Prism stages. (g) Early pluteus seen from the mouth
side. (h) Pluteus seen from the right side. Drawings from a time-lapse film.
The optical sections in (a)–(c) have not passed through the thick plate of
the animal organ (acron). (From Gustafson and Toneby 1971.)

pigment, echinochrome. In connexion with the growth of the skeleton
the larva passes through the so-called prism stage (Fig. 3(l), Fig. 4(f)).
Branches of the triradiate spicules growing in the animal direction later
bend ventrally and participate in formation of the two oral arms on
each side of the animal plate (Fig. 3(l)–(n) *or, oa*; Fig. 5). The ventral
rods grow towards each other and temporarily fuse (ventral transverse
rods, *vtr*). The third rod soon divides into two branches, one growing out
in the anal arm (*ar, aa*), the other in the opposite direction in the part
of the body-wall resembling a pointed cone, the apex (Fig. 5). The rods
may be called the body-rods (*br*). The ciliated band runs from the animal
plate up and down on the arms and across the ventral side, encircling
the oral field (Fig. 5, Fig. 57(a) (see page 113)). The larva has been named
pluteus (Johannes Müller 1846), the Greek name for easel which it
resembles when placed with the front end down. In early papers, and
even in some modern textbooks, plutei are reproduced with this awkward
orientation. Like the blastulae and gastrulae the plutei swim forward
in a spiral.

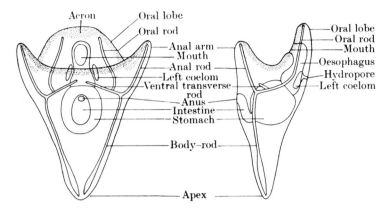

FIG. 5. Diagrams of a young pluteus.

The position of the egg axis in a fully differentiated pluteus larva is indicated by the broken line in Fig. 3(m) (see page 16). The animal pole of the gastrula corresponds to the front edge of the oral lobe (the acron) between the oral arms. The oral field, surrounded by the ciliated band, occupies the greater part of the ventral side. The apex with the two long, thickened body-rods (*br*) represents a part of the dorsal side of the pluteus (Runnström 1928*b*; Hörstadius 1928, p. 67). It is evident that, in comparison to the gastrula, the egg axis has been considerably bent particularly with respect to the oral lobe and the digestive tract.

How is the material used?

Gastrulation is a complicated process which will be dealt with at some length, as an exact knowledge of how different cell layers are used is of crucial importance in the interpretation of experiments. The pigment band in *Paracentrotus* has played a considerable role in the study of the organization of the sea-urchin egg. As early as 1883 Selenka had described the band as a sign of a polar stratification, and attributed it to the vegetal half, but he was in error in considering the mesomeres as vegetal cells. Driesch (1900*a*), on the other hand, discovered that the mesomeres represent animal elements. This result was confirmed by Boveri's (1901*a*, *b*) rediscovery of the pigment ring and description of the pigment-free vegetal cap giving rise to the micromeres. However, he was mistaken in using the pigment to mark the amount of invagination; he had seen that the pigment also reaches a little above the equator, and he states that the whole pigmented region invaginates.

The change from yellow–orange to silver–white of the surface layer of the egg in dark field immediately upon fertilization was described by Runnström (1923) using gametes of *Psammechinus miliaris*. In a later paper (1928*a*) the same reaction was observed with material from three other species, but eggs of *Paracentrotus lividus* gave another picture. The fertilized egg has an orange belt of about the same position as the pigment ring, but the two girdles are not identical as the orange ring exists also in eggs with the pigment equally distributed over the whole surface. At gastrulation the whole orange field was invaginated, even some mesomere material being included in the archenteron.

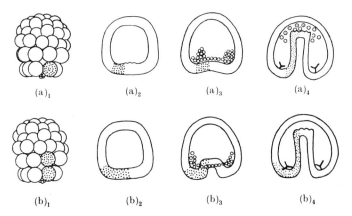

$(a)_1$ $(a)_2$ $(a)_3$ $(a)_4$

$(b)_1$ $(b)_2$ $(b)_3$ $(b)_4$

FIG. 6. Vital staining of single blastomeres and their fate during gastrulation. $(a)_1$–$(a)_4$, *veg$_2$*-cell. $(b)_1$–$(b)_4$, *veg$_1$*-cell and *veg$_2$*-cell. (From Hörstadius 1936*b*.)

von Ubisch had already (1925*a*) stated after local vital staining that the whole vegetal half participates in invagination. This opinion was contested by several authors. Morgan (1895*d*, 1903), Driesch (1902), and Schmidt (1904) estimated from counts of nuclei the invaginating material at between one-tenth and one-quarter of the egg, but for several reasons these counts cannot give decisive results.

As many results of isolations and transplantations were inexplicable on the assumption of an ecto–endodermal boundary an_2–veg_1 a new investigation was made with different methods of vital staining (Hörstadius 1931, 1935, 1936*b*). Groups of blastomeres were stained either by leaning them against agar–agar, or after isolation with subsequent transplantation back to the same position. Staining of veg_2 + the micromeres with Nile blue resulted in a blue colour only being present in the primary mesenchyme and archenteron. Staining of the whole vegetal half showed that about a third of the ectoderm also appeared to be derived from the macromeres. To obtain a decisive answer on this as a basis for future work, single cells of 64-cell stages were stained, using micropipett (see Fig. 8). The staining of one veg_2-blastomere resulted in a blue stripe in the archenteron alone (Fig. 6(a)$_1$–(a)$_4$) whereas marking of both a veg_1-cell and a veg_2-cell showed that veg_1 represents presumptive ectoderm (Fig. 6(b)$_1$–(b)$_4$). The old statements based on the pigment and the shining ring were also tested (Fig. 7). In eggs with a distinct pigment band the granules do not form a sharp line either at the equator or towards the micromeres. A sparse pigmentation may therefore be found on the vegetal side of mesomeres, the more so if the eggs

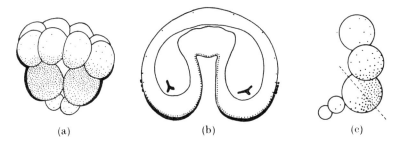

(a)   (b)   (c)

Fig. 7. 16-cell stage (a) and gastrula (b) of *Paracentrotus lividus*. Distribution of the pigment granules, dotted. The heavy lines outside the dotted areas indicate the extent of the layer which in a dark field is shining with a yellow-orange colour. (c) A meridional series of blastomeres from a 32-cell stage. From the animal pole: an_1, an_2, descendant of macromere, large and small micromeres. The furrow that will separate the veg_1- and veg_2-cells indicated by broken line. (From Hörstadius 1935.)

are of the subequatorial type with the third furrow somewhat below the equator. At the veg_1–veg_2-division the furrow cuts through more in a radial direction than parallel to the equator. The veg_1-cells accordingly will receive more of the pigmented surface and will look more strongly coloured (Fig. 7(c)). In the veg_2-blastomeres the granules gradually diminish in number but some may still be found in the micromeres. In the gastrula the pigment is spread over the inside of the archenteron and on the outside of the vegetal ectoderm (Fig. 7(b)) to the same extent as the stain in Fig. 6(b)$_4$ and with only a few granules above the former equator. The pattern of the shining layer in different stages was also controlled: in cleavage stages it embraced not only the macromeres but also the most vegetal part of the mesomeres (Fig. 7(a)), and in the gastrula it covered the same ectodermal area as the pigment (Fig. 7(b)). As a consequence of my preliminary account in 1931, von Ubisch took up his staining experiments again (1933c) and confirmed the findings described in this paragraph.

The prospective significance of the layers an_1, an_2, veg_1, veg_2, and the micromeres in blastula, gastrula, prism larva, and pluteus is shown diagrammatically in Fig. 3(h)–(n).

Two complex processes

The process of gastrulation, that is, the mechanism of invagination, has been the subject of many speculations. The old explanation was that the archenteron material was gradually pushed by the enlarging ectoderm into the blastocoele in the shape of a tube (Boveri 1901a, Fig. 37–39; von Ubisch 1925a; Lindahl 1932c, p. 327). But vital staining showed the following picture. After migration of the primary mesenchyme into the blastocoele the vegetal wall still remains as a fairly thick plate, the presumptive archenteron, which previously formed a ring round the mesenchyme material but is now found as a central disk (Fig. $6(a)_2$, $(a)_3$). From the beginning the invagination affects the whole disk, its wall growing thinner (Fig. $6(a)_3$, $(a)_4$, $(b)_3$, $(b)_4$), obviously without pressure from the surrounding ectoderm (Hörstadius 1935, p. 273, 1936b).

As to the mechanism of invagination, Bütschli (1915) was of the opinion that the inner surface of the endoderm plate would expand more than the peripheral. Spek (1918) showed with an agar–gelatine model that a stronger swelling of the inner layer led to an invagination. In recent years the problem has been thoroughly studied particularly by time-lapse photography (Gustafson, from 1956, literature in Gustafson and Wolpert 1963, 1967). The analysis first disclosed that invagination proceeds in two major steps separated by a short pause. During the first phase the vegetal disk bends inward and forms a more or less hemispherical structure, as in Fig. 4(c). This change of shape is accounted for by the decrease in contact between the cells in this region, associated with pulsatory activity of the cells and a tendency to round up. The cells retain their contact with the hyaline membrane and become pear-shaped. The second phase begins with strong pulsatory activity at the archenteron tip where the future secondary mesenchyme will be budded off. The cells shoot out fine pseudopods which explore randomly and attach to the ectoderm at the junction of ectoderm cells (see Fig. 4(d)). Now they cease extending and instead contract. The further elongation of the archenteron rudiment is said to be the result of contractile activity of these pseudopods (Dan and Okazaki 1956; Gustafson and Kinnander

1956*a*, *b*). It seems surprising that the second part of the invagination should be due only to the pseudopodal pulling. In exogastrulae a similar archenteron is formed in the absence of pulling forces, but here the starting point is different: the process comprises narrowing and stretching of a circular wall without any change of direction.

Contact between the tip of the archenteron and the oral field is brought about after a lively exploration of pseudopods and their subsequent contractile activity (Gustafson and Kinnander 1960).

The primary mesenchyme cells also send out pseudopods for their movements and arrangement in a chain round the base of the archenteron, with stronger concentration to two ventro–lateral clusters (Fig. 3(k), Fig. 4(c, d)). Pseudopods from different cells fuse and a syncytium is formed (Theel 1892; von Ubisch 1937, 1939; Okazaki 1960, 1965). The skeletal granules and rods are formed and grow intra-cellularly, in the pseudopodal syncytium and thus not in the original cell bodies (Theel 1892; von Ubisch 1937; Okazaki 1960). The outgrowth of the rods and the arms as well as the apex depends on interaction between ectoderm and mesenchyme. The position of the skeleton-forming cells is determined by the ectoderm (Herbst 1893, p. 193, 1896; Driesch 1896*a*). Rudiments of arms are predetermined before the skeleton rod reaches the ectoderm but they cannot develop further than as short buds without co-operation with skeleton-forming cells (Jenkinson 1911*a*; MacBride 1914; Runnström 1915). The influence that the skeleton-forming cells exert upon the ectoderm, and which is necessary for the outgrowth of the arms, was called by Herbst 'formativer Reiz' (1892, page 456; 1893, pages 193, 206; 1896; 1897). As a consequence of the predetermination in the ectoderm, arms do not always grow out where a rod reaches the ectoderm (Runnström 1929, p. 131; von Ubisch 1931, 1932*a*, 1933). If a rod is missing another rod may grow towards its place and act as its substitute (Runnström 1928*b*, 1929, 1931). The club-like thickening of a body-rod is only formed in contact with the apex ectoderm. Also oral, anal, and transverse rods may form clubs as by mistake they reach the apical region (Runnström 1931). The statement that apex ectoderm is a prerequisite for formation of body-rods is contradicted by recent cultures *in vitro* of isolated micromeres (Okazaki, pp. 32 and 51).

Moreover, when skeletal rods grow in an atypical way they have a homogeneous crystal structure (Runnström 1931). A time-lapse analysis (Wolpert and Gustafson 1961) has shown that the 'crystallographic mechanism' is responsible for the initial triradiate shape and a tendency of its branches to grow straight. A 'pseudopodal' mechanism is involved in the appearance of angles and in spine formation. The future regions of arm formation can be localized at an early stage by an accumulation of pigment cells. A plug of mesenchyme cells is attached to the skeleton tip. The pseudopods of these cells determine the direction of the rods after random exploration of the ectoderm and preferential attachment to points of strongest adhesion. The ectoderm thus determines the skeletal pattern. The plug of mesenchyme cells causes a tension in the arm ectoderm, resulting in its elongating growth (Gustafson and Wolpert 1961).

The ciliated band consists of cylindrical cells. The greater part of the blastula wall differentiates as a thin squamous epithelium which, however, is somewhat thicker in the oral field. A glance at a late gastrula or a prism larva (Fig. 3(k), (l), Fig. 4(e)) reveals that the ventral side with ciliated band and oral field makes use of more material than the dorsal side with its thin epithelium. The larvae swim forward in a spiral as a result of movements of the cilia in the band. Cilia also bring food particles into the mouth, but further transport through the alimentary canal is brought about by muscular contractions.

In this description of development only the species *Paracentrotus lividus* has been mentioned by name because of the pigment band of the mature egg, but the account is largely also valid for the other commonly used species. *Psammechinus (Echinus, Parechinus) miliaris* and *Psammechinus microtuberculatus* both have skeletons of the same simple type as *Paracentrotus. Sphaerechinus granularis, Arbacia lixula* (formerly *pustulosa*) and *A. punctulata, Lytechinus variegatus, Echinocardium cordatum, Echinocyamus pusillus*, and others, have a more complex skeleton, some of the rods being of the lattice (fenestrated) type (see Fig. 78(b)). In the following discussion the species used will be mentioned only occasionally when the point is of special importance.

4 *Methods*

Sea-urchin gametes: where, when, and how?

THE number of eggs produced by sea-urchins is enormous. It has been estimated that a female *Arbacia lixula* contains about eight million eggs (Harvey 1956). In the much larger *Echinus esculentus* the number reaches 20 million (MacBride 1906). In species with a very short spawning period each animal becomes mature probably only once a year. The reproductive cycles are different in *Paracentrotus lividus*. At Roscoff, in Brittany, the animals have mature sexual products during the summer months. However, in the Mediterranean—for example, at Naples—the material can be obtained throughout the year although winter and spring are the better periods. Practically all animals shed their products during a heavy storm, but after a week or two the gonads are replenished. There is no doubt that the animals of this species acquire sexual maturity several times in a year.

The following list indicates the periods during which usable sexual products can be obtained from the species most commonly used in laboratories in Europe, North America, and Japan.†

Ripe animals of *Paracentrotus lividus* can be found all year round at Naples but the best periods are Feb.–June and Sept.–Nov. At the French station at Banyuls in the eastern Mediterranean (near the Spanish border) spawning is reported from March to July and at Roscoff in Brittany from April to August. *Arbacia lixula* spawns in Naples in

---

† Information on European species has kindly been furnished by Professor J. Bergerard, Roscoff, Dr. D. P. Wilson, Plymouth, and Dr. B. Hagström, Stockholm. The American species are quoted from a list by Hinegardner (1973). Professor H. Kanatani has informed the writer of the species commonly used at Misaki Marine Biological Station. Further data on American and Japanese species as well as of some species off Hawaii have been obtained from Professor G. Czihak, Salzburg.

March, April, August and September and *Spaerechinus granularis* spawns in April, August and September. In Roscoff they are ripe from January to October, but are difficult to obtain in May–July, because sea-urchins can only be collected at extreme low tides. In Naples, *Genocidaris maculata* is ripe from March to June, and *Psammechinus microtuber-culatus* in March, April, May and July. In Roscoff, *Psammechinus miliaris* spawns from April to August, and in Plymouth from May to September. In Bergen spawning is June–August, and in Kristineberg June–August for the Z-form (shallow water) and July–September for the S-form (deeper water). *Echinus esculentus* is ripe in Roscoff in March–June and in Plymouth from the middle of March to the middle of May. It spawns in Bergen in March–May and in Kristineberg in April–May–June. *Echinus acutus* is ripe there in February–March–April, and *Strongylocentrotus dröbachiensis* from the end of February to the beginning of April. *Echinocyamus pusillus* spawns in Bergen in June–September, and *Echinocardium cordatum* in Roscoff in April–August, and in Kristineberg in June–July–September.

On the North-American east coast *Arbacia punctulata* spawns in summer, *Echinarachnius parma* in summer, *Lytechinus variegatus* in winter, and *Strongylocentrotus dröbachiensis* in late winter. On the west coast, *Dendraster excentricus* is ripe in summer, *Lytechinus pictus* in summer, and *Strongylocentrotus purpuratus* from autumn to spring.

From Hawaii are mentioned *Echinometra mathaei*, primarily spawning in winter, and *Tripneustes gratilla* spawning in summer and autumn.

In Japan, the spawning seasons vary somewhat for the same species in the northern and the southern parts. *Hemicentrotus pulcherrimus* spawns in the middle of January–April, *Echinocardium cordatum* in April–July, *Mespilia globulus* in June–September, *Anthocidaris crassi-spina* from the end of June to the beginning of September, *Clypeaster japonicus* in July, *Temnopleurus toreumaticus* in July–August, *Echino-metra mathaei* in July–September, *Peronella japonica* in August, *Astri-clypeus manni* in June–September. In the north, *Strongylocentrotus nudus* spawns in September–November, *Str. intermedius* in October–November, and *Pseudocentrotus depressus* in October–November.

Some species are difficult to maintain in aquaria; others can be kept for long periods and produce gametes even in closed systems far from the sea, provided that several prerequisites are fulfilled. The sea-water must be extremely clean, in closed systems purified by being passed through a coal filter. A strong aeration is imperative: the animals often gather in the region with the stream of air bubbles. The pH can be more or less stabilized by pieces of limestone or shells in the filter but should be controlled occasionally. The temperature must be kept below the upper limit of the temperature range of the species in question. There must be an adequate food supply. Not all species of marine algae are accepted, red algae are often preferred. But sea-urchins can also prosper on salad, shrimps, and boiled fish. Care has to be taken that the water does not become contaminated by food particles.

In several species no sex dimorphism has been detected, for example, in *Arbacia lixula*. In some species the male genital openings are borne on papillae which are missing or shorter in the females (*Echinocyamus pusillus* and *Psammechinus miliaris*, Marx 1929; *Echinus esculentus*, *Psammechinus microtuberculatus*, *Paracentrotus lividus*, *Sphaerechinus granularis*, Swann 1954). In *Lytechinus* the female has larger gonophores than the male (Tyler 1944) and the female pores are surrounded by a dark ring of pigment (Hinegardner 1973). Particularly striking is the dimorphism in the Japanese *Strongylocentrotus pulcherrimus* where on the oral side the male tube feet are white and the female ones yellow (Motomura 1941). For determining the sex in *Arbacia* without opening the animal Harvey (1956) recommends inserting a drop of sea-water saturated with KCl into one genital pore, whereupon eggs or sperm will ooze out from the pore. Alternatively a small amount of material is drawn out with a syringe through a genital pore. According to Hinegardner (1973) the syringe needle can instead be passed through the soft peristomal membrane into the gonad.

There are two different ways of obtaining sea-urchin gametes. The old method is to remove the gonads, the other is to induce spawning. To reach the gonads the peristomal wall of a sea-urchin is removed after a peripheral cut with a pair of scissors. The intestine is taken out. Ovaries with ripe eggs have a brownish or reddish colour, testes are more or less whitish. A pair of curved forceps is gently passed under an ovary, the oviduct is snipped, and the ovary is lifted out and brought into sea-water where it usually starts spawning. From pieces of ovaries greater quantities pour out. As ovarial fluid inhibits fertilization the eggs should be washed twice. In a beaker they soon sink to the bottom and are pipetted off to another glass, or the water may be poured out and renewed. If there is risk of contamination of the urchins by sperm in their aquarium or in the buckets in which they have been brought, it is preferable before opening to dip each animal in a bowl of fresh water which will immediately kill all spermatozoa. In any case scissors and tweezers have to be sterilized in this way after use in a male. As this is easily forgotten it is advisable to form the habit of cleaning both instruments before each dissection.

Spawning has been found to be induced by injection of tissue extract, KCl, or CaCl$_2$ into the body-cavity. Palmer (1935, 1937) and Tyler (1949) recommend the injection of 0·5 ml. of 0·5 M KCl. The animals are then placed with the oral side upwards over a beaker filled with sea-water where they start shedding eggs or sperm. Harvey (1956) has used electric shock for the same purpose (lead electrodes, about 10-volt). It is said that the spawning will stop when the current is turned off. Both the injection and the shock method are liable to hurt the animals.

Most beginners are apt to use far too much sperm in artificial fertilization. Only one or a few drops of the thick white sperm fluid should be added to the sea-water in a beaker—just enough to give the water a light-greyish colour. A few drops of this solution are enough to fertilize a great quantity of eggs. Eggs retain their fertilizability for several hours in sea-water. However, if there is a long time interval between experiments the ovaries should preferably be kept in the shell and new suspensions should be made. The sperm, on the other hand, lose their motility very quickly; new suspensions must be made for each fertilization if the interval exceeds about half an hour. Dry (that is, undiluted) sperm, however, is very stable; it can be stored in a refrigerator for days although the quality may decline.

Operative methods

In studies of unfertilized eggs the jelly layer (Fig. 2) may have to be removed. This is done in acidified sea-water. At a pH of about 4·5, the treatment should last only a few seconds before the eggs are carefully pipetted back to sea-water and again washed (Hörstadius 1936c). At a pH of about 5·5, they may remain in the water for 1–3 minutes (Vasseur 1948; Hagström 1959).

The fertilization membrane is too tough to permit operations to be performed. Several methods have been described for removal of this membrane together with the jelly layer. One way is to prevent the formation of the membrane by pre-treatment with urea, glycerol or proteolytic enzymes. Soon after its formation the membrane can be dissolved by proteolytic enzymes. As eggs treated by such methods cannot be considered normal, mechanical methods are preferable. Driesch (1893b) obtained eggs free of membranes by shaking them shortly after fertilization. Plough (1927) recommends sucking up eggs into a capillary pipette which has a bore of about two-thirds the diameter of the egg membrane. Hörstadius (1935) prefers aspirating the eggs rapidly through a pipette with an orifice three or four times the diameter of the eggs. Hagström and Lönning (1964) found that this procedure can be used also at the 4- or 8-cell stages. Lindahl and Lundin (1948) and Markman (1958) describe devices for gently sucking or pressing the eggs through silk gauze with meshes slightly smaller than the diameter of the eggs. As it is sometimes necessary to test eggs of six or eight females to find which batches fulfil the requirements, the simple and fast aspiration method is probably preferable.

Eggs deprived of a membrane by mechanical means segment and develop further in a normal way if the female has been in good condition and the laboratory environment is suitable. If the eggs are not of good quality—i.e., 80 per cent–90 per cent capable of fertilization—the blastomeres of the 8-cell stage tend to form a ring instead of one quartet on top of the other. The same occurs with good eggs if the temperature is too high. It is imperative to work within the development temperature range of the species which is often narrower than that of the adult. This requirement is a nuisance when dealing, for example, with *Strongylocentrotus dröbachiensis* which requires a maximum temperature of 12°C. Another example worth mentioning is *Paracentrotus lividus*, so commonly used because it can produce gametes all year round in the Mediterranean. However, the summer eggs, accustomed to 26°C, do not segment normally at the winter temperature of the sea, 13°C, and vice versa (Hörstadius 1925*d*).

Another environmental claim: No Smoking. Sea-water rapidly absorbs poisonous substances which preclude normal development. This uncomfortable fact has caused much trouble for beginners unaware of it.

In the early days, blastomeres were isolated by shaking only (Driesch 1891; Fiedler 1891). The discovery by Herbst (1900) that calcium-free sea-water loosens the connexion between blastomeres caused Driesch to use this method before shaking (1902). Zoja (1895) was able to cut cleavage stages, and Jenkinson (1911*a*) blastulae and gastrulae, with a fine knife. Spemann (1906) recommends glass needles for operations on sea-urchin larvae, and such needles are now usually employed on echinoderms (von Ubisch 1925*b*; Hörstadius 1925*b*).

To make fine glass needles a microflame is necessary. The simple device of Spemann shown in Fig. 8(a) consists of a glass pipette with a Hoffman screw clamp on the rubber tube for regulating the gas pressure. As the mouth of the pipette may close because of the heat it is advisable to use the point of a syringe, its oblique opening reduced to a circular one. Micro-burners are also purchasable. A glass rod or tube is melted in a Bunsen flame and drawn out to arms' length to a fine thread. A piece of this thread is drawn out in the microflame. At the same time a quick side movement is made to give the end a curve which makes it more adapted to the operations. A part of the thread with the needle is placed in the microflame and fused with a handle (a rod or tube) from which the thread has been drawn out (Fig. 8(d)).

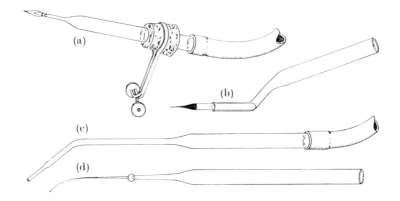

FIG. 8. (a) Microflame (after Spemann 1923). (b) Micropipette for vital staining of single cells (according to Lindahl 1932). (c) Mouth pipette. (d) Glass needle (after Spemann 1923).

Some objects are likely to glide a way from under the needle when placed on glass; for this reason it is preferable to place on the bottom of the shallow operation dish a thin disk of celluloid or other transparent material in which slight grooves have been made by scratching with a pin. It is easier to orient and cut the egg or cleavage stage when they are lying in the groove (Hörstadius 1928). Care should be taken that the material of the disk does not give off any poisonous substances.

For transport of eggs, fragments, single blastomeres, or swimming larvae, a mouth pipette is preferable (Peterfi 1924; Fry 1924). It is hardly possible to keep an ordinary pipette steady when having to regulate the rubber teat with the fingers, and the sucking and aspirating movements will be far too vigorous. A suitable pipette (Fig. 8(c)) is made in the following way. The narrow tube of a fairly long pipette is drawn out a little in the microflame: several attempts may have to be made to obtain the desired dimension of the capillary tube. It is important that the capillary should have a smooth opening; if it is simply broken off it will have jagged edges, so it should be held against a finger-tip and scratched slightly with a diamond before being broken. The pipette is held obliquely in the microflame to obtain an appropriate angle. It is connected by a rubber tube with a mouthpiece consisting of a short glass tube fixed on the dissecting microscope at a height convenient for the lips to reach. Before being used, the pipette should be filled with sea-water by means of capillary force. To pick up a number of larvae, particularly when they are swimming, the use of capillary force is preferable to sucking, which may introduce air bubbles into the pipette and thereby cause trouble. The pipette must be kept extremely clean, otherwise objects may get lost by sticking to the wall: thus it may often have to be renewed—if it does not get broken first. If, after some time, the pipette fails to function the reason may be saliva in the rubber tube. After each day's work the pipette should be cleaned with distilled water, otherwise a plug of crystals may form in the capillary and prove difficult to dissolve. A great advantage of this pipette is that it can be laid on the table, resting in a cut made in the side of a box. When dishes are changed, the objects remain safely close to the mouth of the pipette. Some training is required to avoid sucking or blowing too quickly.

The cleavage cells of some species, such as *Psammechinus miliaris*, can be separated with glass needles without any pre-treatment. In other cases, such as *Paracentrotus lividus*, it is preferable to perform these operations in Ca-free sea-water. Blastomeres of *Arbacia* cannot readily be separated, even in this solution. The blastomeres fall apart if cleavage stages remain too long in the Ca-free sea-water. Care must also be taken that the connexion between cells does not become so loose that the objects cannot tolerate transport in the micropipette back to sea-water without breaking into smaller fragments. The optimal time needed has to be determined; it depends on the species and on the purity of the chemicals used. The finding that the vegetal cells in 32-cell stages stick together more than other blastomeres is explained by the partial breakdown of the cell membranes and fusion of cytoplasm between micromeres and macromeres reported earlier (see page 15).

The following formula for artificial sea-water both for ocean water (35 per mille) and water of the Mediterranean (38 per mille) was published (Hörstadius 1935, p. 263) from calculations by Bialascewicz and by Runnström (1928c).

Number of ml of the solutions		Ocean water (%)	Gulf of Naples (%)
100·0	NaCl	3·29	3·60
2·0	KCl	4·28	4·64
3·5	CaCl$_2$	4·16	4·43
10·5	MgCl$_2$	3·49	3·68
3·0	MgSO$_4$·7 H$_2$O	19·5	21·5
0·1	NaHCO$_3$	5·21	5·21
0·1	NaOH	2·6	2·6

Another formula follows, used in American laboratories (Hinegardner 1973):

	grams per litre
NaCl	28·32
KCl	0·77
MgCl$_2$·6H$_2$O	5·41
MgSO$_4$·7H$_2$O	7·13
CaCl$_2$	1·18

A number of other formulae have been published by Cavanaugh (1956).

For study of the metabolism of different cell layers it has been desirable to isolate great quantities of micromeres, macromeres and mesomeres of 16-cell stages. For this purpose suspensions of disaggregated blastomeres are centrifuged either in a counter-streaming centrifuge (Lindahl and Nyberg 1955) or in a sucrose density gradient. Afterwards the band of cells are removed by pipette (Spiegel and Tyler 1966; Hynes and Gross 1970; Okazaki 1971, 1972). The latter author cultivated isolated micromeres *in vitro*, in sea-water containing 1–2 per cent of horse serum, and obtained skeleton formation (see page 51).

A method of great importance for experimental embryology is local vital staining using pieces of agar (Vogt 1925). A thin sheet of agar is soaked in Nile blue sulphate or neutral red, and washed in several waters until it ceases to give off clouds of stain. As cells take up stain from very dilute solutions this washing is essential. When a small piece is applied against a blastomere the stain diffuses into the cell. The egg is removed when the stain has penetrated about half of the blastomere. The stain will later spread through the entire cell without diffusing into the adjacent cells if the staining has not been too excessive. This method was first used on sea-urchin eggs by von Ubisch (1925a). Another method is to isolate groups of cells, stain them in a solution, wash them, and transplant them back again. In this way it has been possible to stain cell layers in the middle of the body—for example, the an_2-ring (Hörstadius 1935).

For setting very small marks, Lindahl (1932*b*) drew out a capillary tube into a still finer, and short, capillary (5–10 μm in diameter) and broke it off just where it narrowed, by merely pulling it sharply outside the flame: this gave a fine smooth pipette mouth. The capillary tube is broken off about 5 cm from the mouth and this end is closed by melting (see Fig. 8(b)). Such capillaries with only one very fine opening are put into a warm solution of one per cent agar in sea-water with one per cent Nile blue. As cooling proceeds agar will be sucked into the micropipettes. Before use a pipette is taken up and carefully washed. It is important not to keep the pipettes too long in the air as the agar may withdraw from the mouth. The capillary can be inserted into an ordinary pipette which then functions as a holder (Fig. 8(b)), that can be fixed in a micromanipulator before placing the opening with the agar against a blastomere.

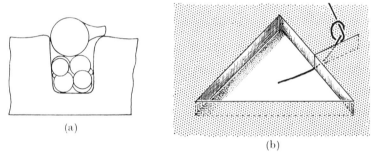

(a)

(b)

FIG. 9. (a) Transplantation of blastomeres. (b) Silk fibre arranged in an agar plate for constriction experiment. (From Hörstadius 1928, 1938.)

For transplantation, fragments are placed one on top of another in a small cylindrical excavation in a transparent plate, like that used for more delicate isolations (Fig. 9(a)). The point of an ordinary pin is beaten against metal until the tip forms a small disk of desired diameter. The pin is screwed down into the plate to a suitable depth. The screwing movement helps to give the cavity a smooth bottom which makes it more transparent and facilitates the orientation of the fragments. A number of pits are made to permit several transplantations at the same time. The fragments coming from Ca-free sea-water are stickier than other cells and are therefore apt to fuse when brought into contact in ordinary sea-water. However, as a rule, a slight pressure is necessary. This is exerted by placing a small glass ball on top of the upper fragment. A fine glass thread, like those used for making needles, is heated in the microflame for a few moments and pulled out quickly, producing an extremely fine swaying thread. The end of this thread is melted in the microflame into a ball slightly larger than an egg and dipped into water. The thread is then broken off with a forceps close to the ball. Pressure should be exerted only for a short while. The larvae must, of course, be transferred to other dishes before they start swimming (Hörstadius 1928).

For constriction experiments a window is cut in an agar plate (Fig. 9(b)). From a silk thread a thin fibre is taken, a loop is made, and the fibre is fixed in a slit of the window wall. A cleavage stage is stuck into the loop which must be of the right size to hold the object, whereupon the loop is slightly tightened by means of two watchmakers' forceps (Hörstadius 1938).

Operations in sea-water are generally performed without sterile precautions.

5 *Determination of cleavage*

THE spindles of the first two cleavages are normally confined to the equatorial plane (Fig. 10(a)$_2$, (a)$_3$). At the next division they are parallel to the egg's axis (Fig. 10(a)$_4$). At the formation of the 16-cell stage, the spindles in the animal quartet again lie perpendicular to the egg's axis (Fig. 10(a)$_5$). Boveri (1901*b*) assumed that consecutive changes in the cytoplasm determine the position of the spindles. It had also been observed that the vegetal cytoplasm has a particular structure (Morgan 1894, for *Arbacia*; Boveri 1901*a, b*, for *Paracentrotus*).

Sometimes whole eggs have been found to segment as fragments (Driesch 1893*a*, 1906; Morgan 1894; Zoja 1895; Boveri 1905, 1910*b*; Hörstadius 1927, 1928). Driesch (1896*b*, 1903, 1906) spoke of an 'anachronism of the furrows' when he saw that eggs in diluted sea-water could form micromeres already in the 8-cell stage (vorzeitige Mikromeren), thus cleaving as a vegetal half (Fig. 10(b)$_5$). Boveri (1905, 1910*b*) obtained half- and quarter-cleavage after shaking the eggs. His explanation was that monasters were formed once or twice—that is, that there were one or two nuclear division cycles without division of the cytoplasm.

Isolated blastomeres of 2- and 4-cell stages as well as groups of 1/8-blastomeres show a partial cleavage as regards the number of meso-, macro- and micromeres (Driesch 1891, 1892; Fiedler, 1891; Zoja 1895, and others) (Fig. 11(a), (b)). Boveri (1901*b*) observed that meridional and vegetal fragments of *Paracentrotus* eggs isolated before fertilization segmented as whole eggs (Fig. 11(c), (e)) while the unpigmented animal fragments gave blastomeres of equal size (Fig. 11(d)). These observations were confirmed on fragments isolated with glass needles and oriented with the aid of the pigment band (Hörstadius 1927, 1928). As early as

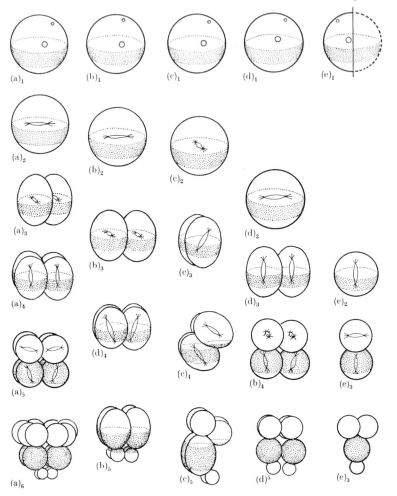

FIG. 10. (a)$_1$–(a)$_6$, normal cleavage of an egg of *Paracentrotus lividus*. Delayed cleavage after shaking or treatment with diluted sea-water leading to formation of micromeres in the 8-cell stage (b)$_5$, or half-cleavage (c$_5$, d$_5$). (e), quarter-cleavage of a meridional half. All stages oriented with vertical egg axis, showing oblique position of many spindles. (From Hörstadius 1927, 1928.)

1896*b* and 1898*b* Driesch obtained fragments of unfertilized eggs by shaking, and he reported in some cases whole, and in some, partial, cleavage.

The results just described provide an explanation as to which factors regulate the cleavage. It is not sufficient to postulate changes in the cytoplasm as governing the position of the spindles and special characteristics of the micromere-forming cytoplasm. In a vegetal half of an

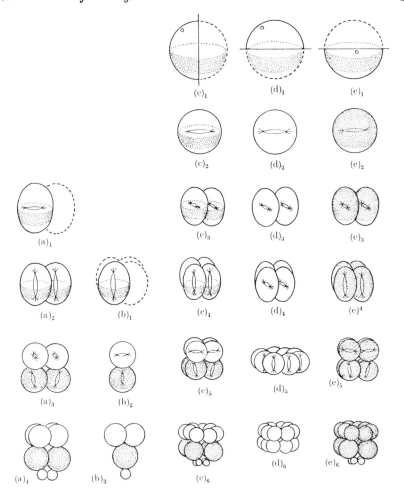

FIG. 11. Cleavage of fragments of eggs of *Paracentrotus lividus*. (a), half-cleavage of half-blastomere. (b), quarter-cleavage of quarter-blastomere. (c)–(e) halves isolated before fertilization. (c), whole cleavage of meridional half. (d), equal cleavage of animal half. (e), whole cleavage of vegetal half.

unfertilized egg, cleaving as a whole, the spindles will have about the same position in the 4-cell stage (Fig. 11(e)$_4$) as in the vegetal blastomeres of egg in the 8-cell stage (Fig. 10(a)$_5$), and yet no micromeres are formed. The vegetal cytoplasm has evidently not yet been activated to form micromeres (Hörstadius 1927, 1928).

The factors determining the cleavage type of the 16-cell stage thus seem to be: first, progressive changes in the cytoplasm which cause spindles formed a certain time after fertilization to lie in a certain direction; second, the presence in the vegetal part of the egg of a region of micromere-forming material; and third, the activation of that material a certain time after fertilization. Fig. 10 shows how it is possible to interpret the partial cleavages of whole eggs by delay (caused by hypotonic sea-water or by shaking) of the nuclear divisions in relation to the progressive changes in the cytoplasm, without assuming monaster formation. This is further supported by the experiment by Painter (1915), who, by means of phenylurethane, inhibited nuclear divisions for some time and afterwards obtained several types of partial cleavage.

Fragments of fertilized eggs also sometimes show whole or partial cleavage (Driesch 1896*b*, Hörstadius 1928). Boveri (1901*b*) opposed Driesch's view that the difference is due to a different faculty of regulation. Boveri instead assumed whole cleavage to occur when the entire surface of the fragment resembles that in the normal egg, while half cleavage would appear when one side is devoid of the normal surface layer. However, Hörstadius (1928, pp. 17, 141) found that meridional halves isolated shortly after fertilization gave whole cleavage, those isolated shortly before first division gave half cleavage, while those in the period between showed intermediate stages (three-quarters cleavage). In this case also the type of segmentation depends upon the time of isolation in relation to the determination process initiated at fertilization.

Morgan and Spooner (1909) concluded from centrifuge experiments that the micromere-forming material is not restricted to the unpigmented area. By removal of fragments of different size it was shown that the material capable of forming micromeres extends up to about the middle of the pigmented region although this capacity gradually decreases. (Hörstadius 1927, 1928).

Of particular interest is the experiment by Driesch (1892 IV, 1893*b*) in which, owing to pressure, the nuclei were atypically distributed in the cytoplasm. Driesch pressed fertilized sea-urchin eggs under a coverslip. In accordance with the rule formulated by Oscar Hertwig (1885) that spindles are formed in the longest axis of the cell body, all blastomeres became spread out in a single layer instead of in rings on top of each other (Fig. 12(a)–(c)). Micromeres could appear in different positions: in Fig. 12(c) they are lying at the edge of the plate. After release of the pressure two layers could be formed. In the egg (d) this led to formation of micromeres in the central part. From the great variety of types of cleavage under pressure and the fact that, irrespective of this variety, plutei developed, Driesch in the first paper drew the conclusion that blastomeres contain equivalent material—they are omnipotent. In the second paper, however, he concisely hit the crucial point by saying that, when each blastomere is capable of producing something other than would result in normal development, he is considering the nuclei, thereby indicating the omnipotency of the nuclei. It is obvious that the nuclei in a flat egg with all spindles in the same plane cannot reach different cytoplasmic regions in the same sequence nor in the same place as in the normal egg with its complicated cleavage pattern. This experiment by Driesch therefore provides the first evidence against the

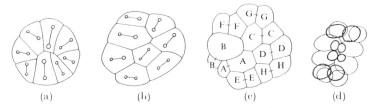

FIG. 12. (a)–(c), cleavage under pressure, all blastomeres and spindles in one layer. In (c) the egg axis is perpendicular to the pressure, with the micromeres to the left. (d), after release of the pressure from a flat 8-cell stage the micromeres formed in central position indicating coincidence of direction of egg axis and pressure. (From Driesch 1892, 1893*b*.)

hypothesis advanced by Weismann (1892) of a distribution of qualitatively different nuclei as the cause of embryonic differentiation.

Driesch knew nothing of the stratification along the egg axis. He therefore could not correctly interpret the stages under pressure. To us it is clear that while the position of the spindles depends on pressure, the egg axis keeps its identity and can occupy any position in relation to the pressure, as shown by the appearance of the micromeres. Micromere formation may be inhibited, for example, by heat or pressure (Driesch 1892), as a result of stretching (Boveri 1901*b*), or of shaking (Hörstadius 1928, p. 124), and yet normal differentiation may occur. Furthermore, plutei may arise from isolated blastomeres showing whole cleavage as well as from whole eggs with partial cleavage; the same is true if the furrows are displaced by pressure or centrifuging. These results indicate that the differentiation of the sea-urchin egg is independent of the type of cleavage that occurs (Boveri 1889, 1895; Driesch 1896*b*, 1898*a*, and others).

The rate of cleavage is not equal in all parts of the egg. In whole eggs the division of the micromeres is delayed in comparison to those of other blastomeres (see page 15). Isolated meso- and macromeres cleave at early stages at almost the same rate, and also at the same rate as do corresponding blastomeres *in situ*. But during the blastula stage the cells of the prospective ectoderm multiply more rapidly than do the cells which later form endoderm and mesoderm (Hagström and Lönning 1964, 1965).

6 *Determination along the egg axis*

WHEN Wilhelm His in 1874 advanced the thesis of organ-forming regions in the egg (organbildende Keimbezirke) he was merely referring to the obvious fact that organs originate in certain parts of the egg. Pioneers of experimental embryology considered that isolated fragments might produce a richer differentiation than that corresponding to the actual fate of the material in normal development. As to the knowledge of the degree of difference between prospective significance and potency, the study of animal and vegetal fragments of sea-urchin eggs has played a considerable and somewhat dramatic role.

In the short introductory historical sketch it was mentioned that Driesch judged the origin of fragments of 8-cell stages from the number of meso-, macro-, and micromeres formed. The lateral and vegetal fragments as well as a minority of animal fragments gastrulated and could more or less develop organs or plutei. On this fact Driesch built his vitalistic philosophy, although the majority of animal fragments remained as blastulae, with enlarged animal tuft. Further support for the harmonious equipotentiality of the cells was provided by the view that the ectoderm in vegetal-half larvae was derived from presumptive endoderm (see pp. 6, 19). However, the findings of Driesch were soon controverted.

In 1895, Zoja isolated animal and vegetal halves with perfect technique by cutting them with minute knives. Their cleavage proceeded as expected. The vegetal halves had no animal tuft, they were ovoid in shape, and the archenteron could form oesophagus, stomach and intestine; whilst none of the animal halves gastrulated, showing instead enlarged animal tuft. Although his results clearly indicated a difference in potency between animal and vegetal material Zoja himself did not

dare to draw the correct conclusion against the authority of Driesch.
He ascribed the lack of gastrulation to unfavourable conditions. Zoja's
results have been confirmed, however, by thousands of cases (Boveri
1901*b*, 1902; Terni 1914; von Ubisch 1925*c, d*; Plough 1929; Hörstadius
in a number of papers 1928–71).

The two main arguments for Driesch's vitalism have thus been
invalidated. The erroneous statement that the whole vegetal half is
endo- and mesodermal has been corrected (see page 20): the use of the
presumptive ectoderm in vegetal halves is further elucidated in this
chapter. The explanation of Driesch's diverging results has already
been given in Chapter 5 by the author's finding that blastomeres after
shaking often segment equally, and then vegetal and meridional fragments may be mistaken for animal (see page 39). In the paper written in
1928, the author (p. 124 of that paper) also isolated animal and vegetal
blastomeres by shaking and obtained about the same percentage of
gastrulating 'animal' fragments as Driesch has reported.

Isolations reveal interactions

The differentiation of isolated animal and vegetal halves is of basic
importance for the study of determination along the egg axis and must
therefore be dealt with at some length. Isolated animal halves present a
number of different types. On the first day after fertilization and operation (in 16- or 32-cell stages) the extent of the animal tuft can vary
considerably, from normal size up to about three-quarters of the surface
(Fig. 13, 3/4–1/8). The next day the stereocilia disappear, and the
blastulae can now be classified into five groups (*A*–*D*). In type *A* the
gastrula is uniformly ciliated; in *Ba* a small part of the wall is transformed
into pavement epithelium; in *Bc* the thin wall extends over more than
half of the surface, the other part remaining as a ciliated field. In *C* a
ciliated band has developed, and in *D* there is moreover a stomodaeum
which is thus formed without any trace of an archenteron being present
(Hörstadius 1935).

In type 1/8 (Fig. 13) the animal tuft indicates the animal pole. The
extension of the tuft might be expected in other types similarly to
follow the meridians, the centre of the thin wall corresponding to the
vegetal pole. This, however, is not the case. A ventro–dorsal organization is discernible, as found by vital staining of the most vegetal cells
of isolated halves (Hörstadius 1936*b*). A tuft (Fig. 13, 1/4) still seems to
have a strictly animal position, but the larger tufts have extended further

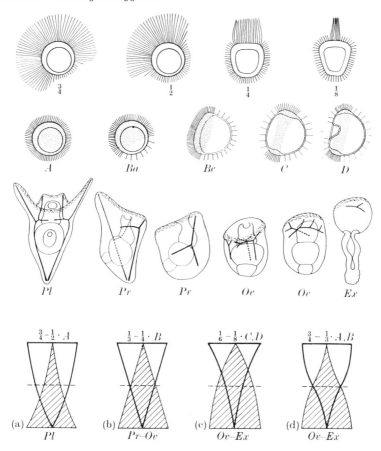

FIG. 13. $\frac{3}{4}-\frac{1}{8}$ classification of animal halves the day after isolation by size of the animal tuft. *A–D*, fully differentiated animal halves. *Pl–Ex*, different types of vegetal halves. *Pl*, pluteus; *Pr*, larvae more or less similar to prism stages; *Ov*, ovoid larvae; *Ex*, exogastrula. The drawings oriented with vertical egg axis. Lowest row: tentative extension of animal (heavy lines) and vegetal (hatched) gradients in relation to observed larval types.

down on the presumptive ventral side (Fig. 13, 1/2, 3/4). This inter-pretation is proved when studying the fully differentiated halves. The ciliated band and stomodaeum in *D* have the proper lateral position in relation to the egg axis. The same applies to the band in *C* which, as a rule, has a broader part representing the most animal region, the acron. The ciliated fields in *Ba* and *Bc* are located in the same angle to the egg axis as the much enlarged tufts.

As indicated by the placing of the drawings in Fig. 13 there is a certain relation between the size of the tuft and the final differentiation. Blastulae with greatly enlarged tuft will mainly give the types *A* and *Ba*, perhaps also *Bc*; the type *D* will be obtained only from blastulae with a small tuft.

The vegetal halves also exhibit a variety of different larval types. They contain only about one-third of the presumptive ectoderm. Nevertheless dwarf plutei may sometimes be found, although as a rule the oral lobe, their most animal part, is somewhat underdeveloped (Fig. 13, *Pl*). In the gastrula stage these larvae may have had an animal tuft, but the great majority of vegetal halves never produce a tuft. The most common type is an ovoid larva (*Ov*). In most cases it has a straight tripartite digestive tract without a mouth, and some irregular spicules under a cap of thick epithelium. Instead of such a ciliated field there may be found in other ovoid larvae a ciliated band encircling an oral field, as a stomodaeum has fused with the oesophagus in forming a mouth. It is striking that the mouth is formed at the animal pole of the half, and that the ciliated band stands at right angles to the egg axis, while in a pluteus both have a lateral position. The larvae between the pluteus and the ovoid larvae in Fig. 13 have been marked *Pr*. This designation stands for types in some respects resembling the prism stage between gastrula and pluteus, as they represent all kinds of intermediate types between ovoid larvae and plutei. The oral field is more or less lateral, the digestive tract more or less curved (cf. Fig. 3(m)), and the skeleton, although often very irregular, has developed spicules some of which can often be identified as oral, anal, or body-rods. An extreme type, on the other side of the ovoid larva, is the exogastrula (Fig. 13, *Ex*).

As an explanation of all the kinds of differentiation of animal and vegetal halves Runnström's concept of two opposite gradients is invaluable. This author deduced from the early isolation experiments and his own findings concerning the action of Li- and K-ions that there exist in the sea-urchin egg two opposite gradients, one animal and one vegetal, both extending from pole to pole and thus overlapping through the whole egg. They interact mutually and are partially hostile to each other as a certain balance is necessary for normal development (Runnström 1928*a*, *b*). This hypothesis was clearly formulated in 1929: 'Wir nehmen zur Eklärung der Determination entlang der Eiachse zwei gegen einander gerichtete und sich gegenseitig beeinflussende Gefälle an . . .' Boveri (1901*b*) had suggested a vegetal gradient. Child, in a number of papers (reviewed 1941), described gradients of susceptibility in echinoderm eggs. But it was primarily the idea of two opposite gradients that has provided the clue to understanding a great number of experimental results.

The enlargement of the animal tuft and the appearance of ciliated blastulae without ciliated band and stomodaeum implies a dominance of animal properties, and, vice versa, the vegetal exogastrula with enlarged archenteron illustrates how vegetal forces have prevailed over animal. Changes of determination in these directions have been called animalization and vegetalization (Lindahl 1933). These terms are preferable to the older endodermization and ectodermization, as—for example—a change of differentiation in vegetal direction not only leads to enlargement of the endoderm and perhaps exogastrulation but also involves inhibition of the animal tuft, displacement of skeleton-forming cells in animal direction, etc. Care must be exercised in the interpretation of observations on changes in development. Exogastrulation is often no sign of vegetalization as lack of invagination can occur without increase in the size of the endodermal region.

Fig. 13 shows the more animal ways of differentiation to the left, and the more vegetal to the right, as regards both animal and vegetal halves. From the drawings of animal halves it can be seen that a certain amount of vegetal influence is necessary to obtain a normal tuft, a ciliated band, and a stomodaeum, otherwise the animal forces will dominate (enlarged tuft, etc.). In the vegetal halves the balance is illustrated by the series of halves retaining sufficient animal properties to contribute to the development of a pluteus, and to an exogastrula in which the ectoderm is much reduced. The correctness of this interpretation is supported by the findings mentioned below.

Before discussing these it must be clearly understood that the occurrence of different types is not due to chance. The eggs within a batch as a rule show a certain limitation of types implying, for example, that within animal and vegetal halves the most extreme animal and vegetal types are rarely found together. The eggs within a batch, therefore, generally can be considered as of animal, vegetal, or intermediate type. A tentative interpretation of the gradients in different cases is given in Fig. 13(a)–(d). Most common are batches with eggs giving intermediate types (b). The results with predominance of animal or vegetal properties are illustrated in (a) and (c). Some batches show the rather puzzling picture of the halves differentiating in different directions (d). It was first believed that the difference was due to the position of the third furrow below the equator as in subequatorial eggs (see page 14) and thus depended on quantity. But later experiments have shown that equatorial eggs also can give pairs of vegetal type. The gradient constitution is the deciding factor. It is only at the end of experiments when the controls are fully differentiated that the type of eggs used can be established. For the sake of simplicity Figs. 15 and 16 are based entirely on results with equatorial eggs which, as has been shown, should rather be termed eggs of animal type.

The distribution of animal and vegetal properties along the egg axis is similar also in the unfertilized mature egg. Animal and vegetal halves were isolated after orientation by means of the pigment band. The animal cells cleaved in the normal way, equally (Fig. 11(d)), while the vegetal halves formed 16-cell stages with meso-, macro-, and micromeres of reduced size (see Fig. 11(e)). Further development resulted in blastulae with enlarged tuft and ovoid larvae (Hörstadius 1935).

In some cases nature itself has separated fragments of unfertilized eggs. A rise in temperature may cause considerable enlargement of polar bodies. Normally these small cells are separated from the egg at the animal pole by a cleavage plane perpendicular to the egg axis (see Fig. 2(b, c), page 11). Lindahl (1937, 1941a) found in eggs of *Strongylocentrotus droebachienses* that the plane by increasing the size of the polar body forms an oblique angle to the egg axis. When the polar body attains the same size as the reduced egg the furrow stands in a meridional relationship to it. After fertilization such twins develop as meridional halves. Gustafson (1946) studied in a more detailed manner the development of twins which were of different sizes and isolated at different angles in relation to the egg axis. Besides plutei, permanent blastulae with enlarged tuft as well as exogastrulae were observed—a proof that animal–vegetal stratification was already present at the time of the maturation process.

The indispensability of vegetal influences for obtaining a normal differentiation of animal material has been studied by experiments which impede the flow of active substances from the vegetal half. According to Lindahl (1932b, 1936, p. 187) a stretching along the egg axis is sufficient to cause an enlargement of the animal plate. Early equatorial constriction by means of a silk fibre (Fig. 14) also leads to enlarged tuft and prevents the formation of ciliated band and stomodaeum, even where the oesophagus extends up into the animal half (Fig. 14(a)$_1$, (a)$_2$). In (b) the most animal third of the embryo is partly isolated by the constriction: both band and stomodaeum are lacking. Instead by a regulatory mechanism they have been formed in the vegetal part. In (c) the animal part has band but no stomodaeum. The real proof is given by constriction in later stages. In $(d)_1$ only a loose silk-loop is laid at the cleavage stage. In spite of tight constriction at a late blastula stage $(d)_2$ the animal half $(d)_3$, secondarily fallen apart from its vegetal partner $(d)_4$, possesses both band and stomodaeum. The necessary interactions have evidently taken place before severance of the connexion. The vegetal half exogastrulated as many vegetal halves do. In (e) the vegetal influences have also reached the animal part before the late constriction.

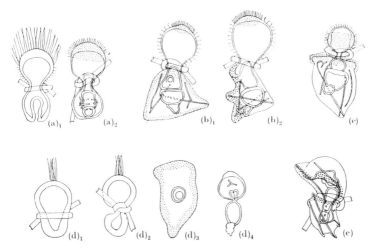

FIG. 14. (a)–(c), equatorial constriction at early cleavage stage. At a late blastula stage the originally loose silk-loop $(d)_1$ has been more tightly constricted $(d)_2$, (e); $(d)_3$, $(d)_4$, the animal and vegetal halves of d_2 (fallen apart). (From Hörstadius 1938.)

The larva resembles a pluteus with a narrow belt and undersized rods: compare the poor differentiation of the animal material in (a), (b) after early constriction. It is less probable that the inhibition is due to closure of the opening between parts of the blastocoele than to the very attenuated cell-wall connexions.

Isolations combined with transplantations

An analysis by means of isolations and transplantations of transverse regions (Fig. 15, 16) shows how dependent the determination and differentiation processes are upon interactions between layers possessing animal and vegetal properties in varying degrees.

First we may compare the development of an animal half (Fig. 15(a)) with that of a half to which, by a section between veg_1 and veg_2, is added the adjacent veg_1-ring, $8+veg_1+0$ (Fig. 15(b))—that is, a larva still

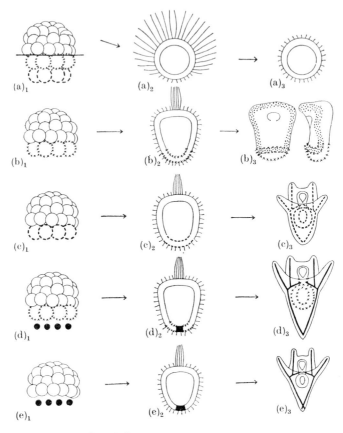

FIG. 15. Diagram of the influence of veg_1, veg_2, and the micromeres on the differentiation of 'equatorial' animal material. an_1 and an_2, continuous lines; veg_1, crosses; veg_2, broken line; micromeres, black. (a), isolated animal half. (b), $8+veg_1+0$. (c), $8+veg_2+0$. (d), $8+veg_1+4$. (e), $8+0+4$. (From Hörstadius 1935, 1939.)

consisting of only ectoderm material, in fact the entire presumptive ectoderm. Its development is quite different from that of an animal half. The tuft is normal, and the larva has a ciliated band and mouth. The region below the equator, although ectodermal, evidently contains more vegetal properties than does the animal half: these have been able to inhibit the extension of the animal tuft and, together with the animal material, bring about the differentiation of ciliated band and stomodaeum. In Fig. 15(c) a veg_2-ring has been fused with an animal half. The larva consists of two-thirds of the ectoderm material and the whole presumptive archenteron. The occurrence of a tripartite digestive tract consequently accords with expectations—exceeded, however, by this endoderm material. It has not only checked the extension of the tuft and induced ciliated band and stomodaeum but has also produced skeleton-forming cells. This implies the formation of cells of more vegetal character than their prospective significance. While the effect on the animal half is an action at a distance, the appearance of the new skeleton-forming cells involves a transformation of part of its material to another task. In terms of two gradients the veg_2 has enhanced the vegetal properties in the animal half, and moreover given its own most vegetal region a greater concentration of vegetal forces than it ever had before.

Implantation of four micromeres into presumptive ectoderm, $8+veg_1$ $+4$, $8+0+4$ (Fig. 15(d), (e)) reveals that the micromeres have the same inhibiting and inductive power as was found in veg_1 and veg_2. Normally they produce the primary mesenchyme cells which secrete the spicules. This is also true in the present instance, but, in addition, they convert the adjacent presumptive ectoderm to archenteron. The result will be a pluteus (provided that the micromeres have been implanted into the most vegetal part of the host). In $8+0+4$ the digestive tract is often proportionately a little too small.

The question arises whether the micromeres maintain their function of forming primary mesenchyme or participate in forming the archenteron. When the micromeres were vitally stained before implantation it was found that in some larvae all their descendants migrated into the blastocoele as primary mesenchyme. In other larvae a little blue material remained in the blastula wall and was found at the tip of the archenteron. Counting of the primary mesenchyme cells pointed in the same direction. In some larvae the normal number, 50–60 (*Paracentrotus*), was found; in other larvae the number was somewhat reduced (Hörstadius 1935, p. 331).

Fig. 15 thus illustrates the increase in vegetal properties that occurs towards the vegetal pole, but some details must be added. The potencies of inhibiting the extension of the animal tuft and of bringing about the differentiation of ciliated band and stomodaeum seem to begin near the equator. At the level veg_1–veg_2 are generally to be found the upper limit of the endoderm-forming material and—a little further down—that of the skeletogenous material. This is shown by the fact that $8+veg_1+0$ of subequatorial eggs may form a small archenteron and sometimes also spicules (Hörstadius 1931, 1935, p. 323; von Ubisch 1933, p. 63). The latter indicates a reconcentration of vegetal forces similar to that of skeleton formation in $8+veg_2+0$. Finally, the material below the presumptive endoderm, the micromeres, can induce endoderm.

Another case of reconcentration at a new pole is provided by the appearance of animal tuft in larvae from which the an_1-ring has been removed, as well as in some vegetal halves (see page 44).

The gradual changes in the system along the egg axis is further evidenced by a study of isolated layers (Fig. 16): an_1 is covered all over with long immovable cilia, a more animal differentiation than isolated halves ever show. The final stage is a ciliated blastula, resembling type A

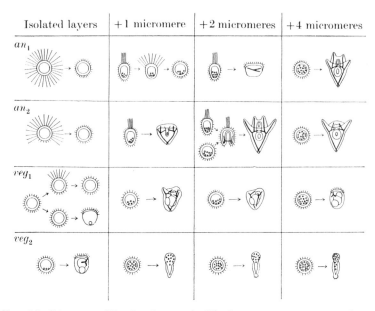

Isolated layers	+1 micromere	+2 micromeres	+4 micromeres
an_1			
an_2			
veg_1			
veg_2			

FIG. 16. Diagram of the development of the layers an_1, an_2, veg_1, and veg_2 isolated (left column), and with 1, 2, and 4 implanted micromeres. (From Hörstadius 1935.)

(see Fig. 13*A*). an_2 behaves just like an animal half of animal type, the stereocilia covering about three-quarters of the surface. The development of veg_1 is particularly interesting as it may follow two lines. On the first day after operation these fragments did not form any such tuft as might be expected of this material from below the equator. However, apparently a kind of contest between the gradients was going on, each struggling to lead the differentiation in its own direction. In some blastulae the animal faculties managed to reconcentrate to form a tuft, whereupon the development proceeded in animal direction towards ciliated blastula. Other blastulae, however, developed no tuft. Instead the vegetal forces succeeded in asserting themselves by invaginating a very small archenteron. A good example of regulation in the form of reconcentration at both ends is offered by veg_2: the ectoderm of the ovoid larva is a more animal differentiation, the skeleton a more vegetal differentiation, than that of the material—presumptive endoderm. (Hörstadius 1935.)

Driesch (1900*a*, p. 375) mentions that one micromere, isolated by shaking, forms a heap of ten cells, nothing more: he doubts whether it can be called a blastula. von Ubisch (1931, p. 197) confirms the statement by Driesch that isolated micromeres (probably groups of four micromeres) form blastulae. Hörstadius (1935, p. 367, *Paracentrotus*) found that isolated groups of micromeres formed 'blastulae', but only if during the cleavage stages they had several times been detached from the bottom. Later they became dissolved into a heap of free rounded cells of about the same number as primary mesenchyme cells. The micromeres therefore seem to be so strongly vegetal that a reorganization to a more harmonious larva is impossible. In studies of isolated single micromeres (Hagström and Lönning 1969, *Echinocyamus pusillus*) no blastulae were observed. Instead, the cleavage pattern was characterized by the temporary occurrence of a syncytium with blunt pseudopodia. One micromere could be reared to form more than 20 cells spread out on the bottom.

The culture of isolated micromeres *in vitro* in a medium consisting of 1–2 per cent horse serum in sea-water has, however, shown that micromeres without any contact with other cells are capable of skeleton formation (Okazaki 1971, 1972, and personal communication). The isolated micromeres first divided unequally, as they do *in vivo*. The further divisions occurred in two different ways. Either the cell membranes became invisible, as in syncytia, or they remained discernible throughout the cleavages. After these divisions the cells appeared to fuse, forming a cell mass; but within a few hours the contour of each cell again became clear, the cells being then designated a cell aggregate. Both cell masses and cell aggregates were capable of coalescing into larger masses or aggregates. If the cells of aggregates dispersed, sometimes showing an arrangement similar to a mesenchymal ring, no spicules were formed. In the remaining aggregates spicules developed at the centre, either as a small rod which probably could give rise to only a two-dimensional skeleton, or as triradiate spicules growing into three-dimensional skeletons. Following the growth of a spicule, cells began to separate from the aggregate, sending out pseudopodia. The three-dimensional skeletons were very similar to the skeletons of

normal plutei both in shape and size and showed species specificity.
Thickened ends of body-rods appeared, thus without influence from an
apex ectoderm, and other rods remained simple or became fenestrated,
according to the pattern of the species.

So far reduction of material has been achieved by removing cell
layers from whole eggs or by isolating small fragments. Another method
of reduction is to suck out central cytoplasm before fertilization by
means of a micropipette in a micromanipulator (Hörstadius, Lorch, and
Danielli 1950). Even when the total cytoplasmic reduction amounted
to 50 per cent the resulting plutei were normal in every respect except
size. The loss did not prevent reorganization into a typical gradient
system. Dalcq (1941) has suggested that the animal gradient might be
cortical and the vegetal located in the interior. The findings do not accord
with this view as harmonious larvae developed, although the ratio of
cortex to central cytoplasm altered considerably.

The interplay between the gradients was further clarified by implantation of 1, 2, or 4 micromeres in isolated an_1–veg_2-layers (see Fig. 16).
One micromere in an_1 was capable of checking the extension of the tuft.
With a normal tuft and some primary mesenchyme in the blastocoele a
small pluteus could be expected as a result of the development. However,
the reorganization of the gradient system was not completed. On the
following day the animal forces took the lead, causing enlargement of
the tuft and suppression of the tendencies to form archenteron and skeleton. Two micromeres managed to keep the tuft in check and to produce
skeletal spicules, but they were not strong enough to induce an archenteron. With 4 micromeres a patently typical balance was attained, resulting in a pluteus. In Fig. 16 an_2 offered less resistance to the vegetal
implant. Already 1 micromere could exert all the expected influence, but
the archenteron became very small. The most harmonious differentiation was obtained with 2 micromeres, while 4 micromeres produced
plutei more like those from vegetal halves.

The similarity of different types of vegetal halves was pronounced in
all cases of implantation in veg_1. Veg_1+4 seems to have the same
constitution as veg_2+0. The vegetal constitution of veg_2 is so strong
that even as little as one micromere causes exogastrulation. With an
increasing number of micromeres the exarchenteron became larger and
the ectoderm smaller.

Fig. 16 illustrates what has been called 'the battle between the animal
and vegetal forces.' In an_1+1 the struggle and the defeat of the vegetal
power can be followed. The other combinations provide a pattern of

different types of balance between the contending tendencies. The further from the animal pole, the less is the resistance to the vegetal influences. This gradual diminution is particularly striking in the context of the search for those larvae that give the most harmonious differentiation. They are found in the diagonal an_1+4, an_2+2, veg_1+1, veg_2+0.

One of the first transplantations made was a fusion of an animal half with a meridional half (Fig. 17) (Hörstadius 1928, p. 76, 1935, p. 349). The polarity of the halves are at right-angles to each other. The micromere region is in close contact with an_2-material. If the animal half has

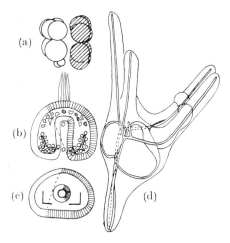

FIG. 17. Fusion of a meridional half with a vitally stained animal half (hatched). See text for further explanation. (From Hörstadius 1935.)

been stained the tuft is placed not far from the margin of the blue ectoderm, and about one-third of the archenteron consists of stained material. This means, first, that a new egg axis is formed, a compromise between the two halves and, second, that the vegetal material of the meridional half has converted adjacent presumptive ectoderm to endomesoderm. This transformed material reaches to the top of the archenteron where it also contributes to the secondary mesenchyme, as some of its cells were stained (Fig. 17(b)). The amount of induced endoderm may be estimated at about one-third of the archenteron, as seen from the optical transverse section (Fig. 17(c)). The dots on the inside of the other part represent red pigment granules of the presumptive endoderm. Larvae with this type of constitution develop into plutei (Fig. 17(d)), thus illustrating a perfect regulation as regards both animal–vegetal and ventro–dorsal organization.

The outcome of the last-mentioned experiment, with endodermization of presumptive ectoderm in contact with the most vegetal material and consequent appearance of a new animal–vegetal axis, may lead to the question of what happens when a meridional half develops into a pluteus. Driesch put the question as early as his first Entwicklungs-mechanische Studien, in 1891. It has been shown that an isolated half-blastomere segments as a half-egg (see Fig. 1 and Fig. 11). At later

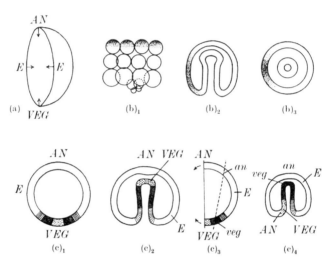

FIG. 18. (a), diagram of closure of a meridional half. $(b)_1$–$(b)_3$, vital stain-ing of the most-animal material of a meridional half, and its position in the gastrula. Diagram of the archenteron material in a late blastula $(c)_1$, in a gastrula $(c)_2$, and in a meridional half-gastrula $(c)_4$. AN, VEG, position of the animal and vegetal pole material in a whole larva $(c)_1$, $(c)_2$ respectively in a meridional half $(c)_3$, $(c)_4$. an, veg, the pole material in a meridional half. The broken line in $(c)_3$ indicates the position of the an–veg axis of a half in relation to the original egg axis. (From Hörstadius 1928, 1935.)

cleavage stages it forms an open half-sphere. Driesch asks whether at closure poles and equator subsist, or not. In the one case, E in Fig. 18(a) would fuse with E, which means maintenance of polarity and stratifica-tion. In the second case a problem arises as to how the material is to be used. Driesch in his first paper is inclined to believe in the solution EE, but in a later paper (1906) he inclines towards the interpretation $EANEVEG$.

Vital staining of the animal pole proved that the marginal material from all sides endeavours to meet in one point, with the result that most animal and most vegetal cells meet (Fig. 18(b)$_1$–(b)$_3$). This disrupts the whole organization. How will the material be used? In accordance with the result illustrated in Fig. 17, endodermization of the cells lying close to the strongest vegetal region would be expected, but this did not occur. The archenteron consists only of presumptive endomesoderm. However, the process of invagination indicates that its material has been used in a different way; the tip contains stomach material and the presumptive oesophagus has contributed to the intestine (Fig. 18(c)$_1$–(c)$_4$). At the same time the direction of the egg axis has been slightly shifted. In meridional halves where the proportions of the layers are normal the larva has evidently preferred to perform the reorganization within the original strata, without trespassing on new adjacent areas. One reason for this may be that most animal material, now in contact with the vegetal pole, is particularly difficult to endodermize, as is shown by several of the following experiments.

The induction power of micromeres and the increasing animal resistance along the egg axis are also demonstrated by lateral implantation of vitally stained micromeres at different levels of whole eggs.

Implantation of a group of 4 micromeres between an_2 and veg_1 (Fig. 19(a)$_1$) has a double effect. Their descendants migrate in the usual way as primary mesenchyme into the blastocoele, but they do not move to join the mesenchyme ring of the host. Instead, the micromeres have induced a new centre attracting the mesenchyme (a)$_2$. Here also an invagination starts, but this second archenteron is smaller than that of the host (a)$_3$. As the invaginations are so close to each other they eventually fuse. Likewise, the groups of mesenchyme cells join and by a regulating mechanism form a typical pair of skeletal rods, the end result being a typical pluteus (a)$_4$.

Different results are obtained by placing the micromeres between an_1 and an_2 (Fig. 19(b)$_1$). The induction of a new vegetal centre will again be observed, guiding the mesenchyme (b)$_2$ and performing an invagination, but in this case both retain their individuality. The archenteron is smaller than in the experiment just described; it does not fuse with that of the host, but differentiates into stomach and intestine. The skeleton formation may lead to a double set, a smaller pair belonging to the induced archenteron (b)$_3$. Alternatively, a new skeleton piece is formed only on one side, the one piece of the host serving as partner also to the intruder.

The first effect of implantation in the animal pole (Fig. 19(c)$_1$) is a complete inhibition of the animal tuft. The further differentiation

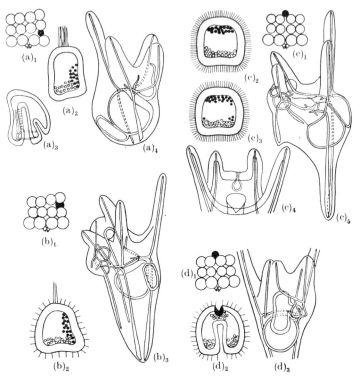

Fig. 19. Implantation of four micromeres into a 32-cell stage; (a) between its animal and vegetal half, (b) between an_2 and an_1, and (c) into the animal pole. (d) implantation of veg_2-cells into the animal pole. (From Hörstadius 1935.)

demonstrates the increasing resistance to induction. Also common to all larvae is a concentration of the vitally stained primary mesenchyme, or at least the majority of the cells at the animal pole $(c)_2$, $(c)_3$. A few have been attracted to the host centre in the larva $(c)_3$. The final differentiations varied widely, indicating that the adjustment to a new equilibrium of the gradients could proceed in different ways. In one larva two spicules but no archenteron were found. After about two days the spicules became smaller and disappeared: the implant had been defeated. In some larvae spicules remained, but the implant could not bring about an invagination. In other plutei, however, a very small invagination was found right in the animal pole, but no spicules were noted $(c)_4$. Several plutei had both archenteron and skeleton reminiscent of the larvae in experiment (b), but now obviously at the top of the oral lobe $(c)_5$. In one pluteus the normal mouth failed to appear; instead, the small induced archenteron developed an opening in the oral lobe, thereby establishing a small digestive tract with reversed polarity. The results illustrate how the intruding vegetal forces have difficulty in asserting themselves in the most animal region, the struggle yielding different examples of new equilibria, including complete defeat.

In the larva Fig. 19(d) two veg_2-blastomeres were implanted in the animal pole. The blastula had a tuft which, however, was somewhat laterally displaced. In the experiments just described the implant migrated into the blastocoele as mesenchyme and the surrounding presumptive ectoderm converted into invaginating endoderm. In our

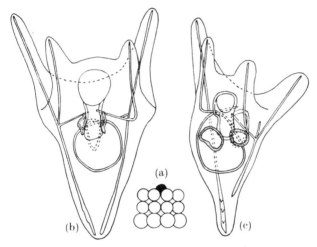

FIG. 20. The micromeres transplanted from the vegetal to the animal pole of the same egg (a). As compared to the control larva (b), the digestive tract and particularly the coeloms are enlarged at the expense of the ectoderm (c). (From Hörstadius 1935.)

case it is the vitally stained presumptive endoderm that forms the archenteron $(d)_2$. This becomes surrounded by a ring of primary mesenchyme cells, attracted from the other pole—a clear illustration of the fact that the position of the primary mesenchyme depends upon stimuli from the wall (compare page 23). Two supernumerary spicules were formed: the archenteron became bipartite and fused with the oesophagus $(d)_3$.

Of interest in this context is the differentiation of a larva of *Psammechinus miliaris* in which the micromeres were removed and implanted in the animal pole (Fig. 20(a)). The vegetal gradient was weakened by the loss of the micromeres at the vegetal pole. Simultaneously, the animal gradient was weakened by the micromeres added to the animal pole. Here they did not cause any induction of the type already discussed. No invagination took place. Only a few primary mesenchyme cells were attracted to the site of implantation; the majority went to the vegetal pole. A pluteus ensued (c). A comparison with a control pluteus (b) reveals the following. The ectoderm is smaller than in the control, and the stomach is larger in outline. Considering that the stomach wall is also thicker, it is evident that the operated larva contains much more endoderm. Most striking, however, is the size of the coeloms. In the control they are typical for this stage: small thin-walled vesicles with very little lumen. In our larva there were two large vesicles with abnormally thick walls. The weakening of both gradients in this case led to a new balance which permitted an increase in endoderm and mesoderm. The author has observed plutei of similar type, with enlarged coeloms, after endodermizing action of lithium in low concentration.

Implantation of 4 micromeres into the animal pole of an animal half yielded varying, and partly unexpected, results. The implantation was not altogether easy: there seemed to be a tendency of the micromeres to move down towards the vegetal part of the half (cf. Fig. 26). In order to ensure a proper implantation the micromeres were stained with neutral red and the animal part of the an_1-material with Nile blue (Fig. 21(b)). A second control was carried out by noting the presence in some halves of the red pigment granules on the vegetal side (dots outside the wall, (b). The first observation concerns the animal tuft. The micromeres prevented its outgrowth in the animal pole but did not completely inhibit its appearance. The tuft was, so to speak, pushed away instead. In Fig. 21(d)$_1$ it is found in a lateral position; in (c)$_1$ it forms a girdle.

The second observation deals with the primary mesenchyme. As might be expected, cells congregate at the induced centre at the animal pole, but another group has migrated down to the vegetal end of the blastula (c)$_1$, (d)$_1$. The ectoderm here, originating from just above the equator, in these larvae also has a power of attraction. Both these opposite groups are able to produce spicules (c)$_1$, (d)$_1$, (e). Invagination showed the greatest variation. In some larvae it failed to occur. In other cases an archenteron was induced at the animal pole, as expected (d)$_2$. It is remarkable to find two invaginations in some larvae (c), as the experience from isolation of thousands of animals halves has proved their inability to gastrulate. The explanation must be that the micromeres in the animal pole so weakened the animal gradient that the vegetal

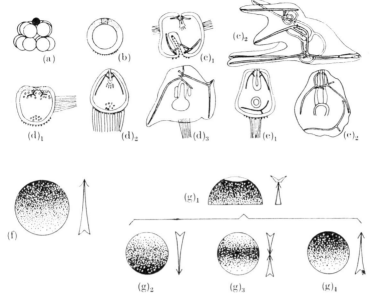

FIG. 21. Implantation of four micromeres (black in (a), hatched in (b)) into the animal pole of an animal half. (b) Checking the site of implantation by use of two vital stains. (c)$_1$, (c)$_2$ Larvae with two archenterons, one induced at the animal pole, and one, the larger, invaginated from the most vegetal side of the animal half. The animal tuft in (c)$_1$ shows that the most animal region is now situated between the two vegetal centres, cf. also (d)$_1$. (d), (e) Reversal of the polarity, archenteron only at the animal pole. (f), (g) Diagrams to illustrate the changes in the gradient system (animal gradient black, vegetal white) as well as the polarity (arrow indicating at the same time polarity and the vegetal gradient). (f) Normal egg. (g)$_1$ Immediately after implantation. (g)$_2$ Reversal of polarity as in (d), (e). (g)$_3$ Two opposite systems as in (c). (g)$_4$ When the original vegetal gradient takes the lead. (From Hörstadius 1935, 1950b.)

gradient in the vegetal region of the half was strong enough to cause an invagination.

A gradual regulation within the gradient system could be followed in larvae with only a single (animal) invagination. In Fig. 21(d)$_1$ the tuft is displaced to the side. Two spicules lie at the site of invagination, and a chalk granule is found at the opposite end, a token of a weak vegetal centre. It was remarkable that the tuft disappeared from the side and reappeared at the presumptive vegetal side, as if it were moving down to the new position (d)$_2$. Simultaneously the granule was dissolved, the small archenteron tied off **t**wo coelomic vesicles and fused with a stomodaeum, and the skeleton grew out as shown in (d)$_3$. These features together illustrate a progressive reorganization of the gradient system leading to a reversal of the polarity. Another example is shown in (e). In this larva the archenteron was larger. The single spicule in the new animal region did not become resorbed.

Summarizing the results we note that differences in strength of the host system as well as of the micromeres lead to different reactions. The host can for the most part maintain its polarity but allow skeleton formation in its animal region also. Only one larva was found in which a vegetal invagination alone took place $(g)_4$. At the new centre in most cases an archenteron and a pair of spicules can be formed. The same processes may occur simultaneously at the opposite pole because the animal faculties have been weakened by the implantation $(g)_3$. The result will be twins of opposite polarity within the same skin $(c)_2$, $(g)_3$. Finally the new centre may completely subdue the surrounding animal forces and cause a reversal of the egg axis $(d)_3$, $(e)_2$, $(g)_2$.

Quantitative relationships

A gradual diminution of vegetal material shed further light upon the interactions in early larvae. Driesch (1893a) found that fragments without micromeres could produce plutei. This statement was confirmed by removing the micromeres from whole larvae (Hörstadius 1928, p. 80; Plough 1929; von Ubisch 1931b, p. 195). It is also clear from the experiment $8 + veg_2 + 0$ reported on page 48 that the skeleton-forming capacity is not restricted to the micromere region (see Fig. 15). The question arises how and when this reconcentration to the most vegetal function occurs. No primary mesenchyme was formed before invagination in larvae deprived of micromeres, but as soon as the archenteron had invaginated half-way, mesenchyme cells were released from the tip. They moved down and gradually formed a ring around the base as well as two groups of spicules. Not only the formation of the cells but also their arrangement in rings and groups implied a considerable delay in development. From this it may be concluded that the regulation involving re-creation of cells capable of skeleton formation as well as their arrangement is not an instantaneous affair but requires some time (Hörstadius 1935, p. 318).

When two macro- and two micromeres are removed from an embryo the result is nevertheless a typical pluteus (Fig. 22(a)). It is, however, impossible to judge with certainty if the proportions of ecto–endoderm are the same as in a normal larva. Two digestive tracts may have the same circumference, but if the walls of the one are thinner it may contain much less material. In a pluteus $8 + 2 + 0$ the skeleton is secreted by

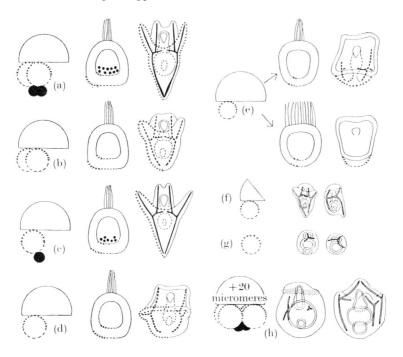

Fig. 22. Diagram of gradual diminution of vegetal material (a)–(e). Animal half, half-circle; veg_1, crosses; veg_2, broken line; micromeres, black. (a) $8+2+2$. (b) $8+2+0$. (c) $8+1+1$. (d) $8+1+0$. (e) $8+\frac{1}{2}+0$. (f) If the animal material is correspondingly diminished, this small larva will differentiate harmoniously, as the animal and vegetal qualities are more typically balanced. (g) If the animal material is removed the half-macromere will differentiate in a much more vegetal way. (h) If a whole egg is filled with micromeres, it will differentiate like a vegetal half. (From Hörstadius 1935, 1936b, 1939a.)

cells formed after a regulation to more vegetal capacity (b). The larvae $8+1+1$ (c) undoubtedly have too small a digestive tract but a well-developed skeleton. Larvae $8+1+0$ are poorly developed regarding both endoderm and skeleton (d). A glance at (a)–(d) reveals that the skeleton is always better developed when formed by its proper material, from micromeres.

In $8+\frac{1}{2}+0$ (e) the same unstable balance may be observed, the same struggle that has been noted in isolated veg_1-rings (see Fig. 16). In some larvae the animal tuft is still of normal size and both archenteron and skeleton appear, but both are very poorly developed. In other cases the vegetal forces in the half-macromere have not been able to hold their own against the animal pressure. The tuft has enlarged and the power of mesenchyme and endoderm formation is completely suppressed.

It is possible to prove, by reducing the presumptive ectoderm to the same degree (Fig. 22(f)), that the vegetal faculties in the veg_2-material of a half-macromere taken by themselves are sufficient to combine into a harmonious whole (f). If only the proper animal–vegetal balance is restored plutei smaller than one-eighth of an egg can develop (compare also Fig. 48). A strange exception to this rule was found when working with the experimental series of Fig. 15. The presumptive ectoderm, $8+veg_1+0$, passes a stage with normal tuft to form blastulae with ciliated band and stomodaeum (Fig. 15(b)). With 'subequatorial'

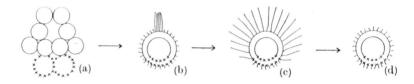

FIG. 23. While $8+veg_1+0$ larvae always develop a normal tuft as well as ciliated band and stomodaeum (see Fig. 15(b)$_2$, (b)$_3$, the animal forces unexpectedly completely dominate in meridional quarters (a) of the same constitution, $(8+veg_1+0)/4$. (b) Early blastula with normal tuft. (c) Older blastula with much extended tuft. (d) Fully differentiated ciliated blastula of animal type. (From Hörstadius 1939a.)

eggs a small invagination and spicules may appear. Meridional quarters of $8+veg_1+0$ always first developed a normal tuft, as expected, but soon afterwards the tuft became very much enlarged, and the fragments developed only into ciliated blastulae (Fig. 23), thus resembling the animal halves of the most animal type (see Fig. 13 (3/4, A) and Fig. 15(a). This is not because the fragments are too small to differentiate, as four more vegetal fragments of the same size $((an_2+4+0)/4)$ gave plutei, and our larvae (Fig. 22(f)) are still smaller. Nor is it due to qualitative differences between dorsal and ventral, since both right and left halves of $8+veg_1+0$ develop into blastulae with ciliated band stomodaeum. Thus the vegetal forces in veg_1, when quantitatively below a certain level, cannot resist the animal ones, although their relative amounts are the same as in the entire $8+veg_1+0$ (Hörstadius and Wolsky 1936). So far we know of no explanation of this phenomenon.

Isolated half-macromeres, without additional presumptive ectoderm, lead to formation of ovoid larvae (Fig. 22(g)).

In another experiment the vegetal forces were increased by implantation of several groups of micromeres into a whole egg (Fig. 22(h)). This also led to a development like that occurring when vegetal halves differentiate into ovoid larvae (see Fig. 13 (*Ov*)).

Strange reactions to rearrangements

Implantation of micromeres into the vegetal or the animal pole of animal halves has led to considerable changes in the gradient system (see Fig. 15(e), and Fig. 21). In all cases the effect has been produced along the original egg axis. In Fig. 17 the axis may be seen as a compromise between two halves at right-angles to each other. Micromeres in lateral positions in whole embryos have induced new, short axes (see Fig. 19). A further study of larvae composed of parts with their egg axes at different angles to each other has revealed the following.

When a meridional half by transplantation is rotated through 90° in relation to the other half, two archentera are invaginated but we then observe the same phenomenon as in larvae with micromeres between an_2 and veg_1—namely, that the archentera move towards each other and fuse. The larvae assume the shape of a pluteus but the skeleton may be somewhat irregular, the bilateral symmetry having been incompletely adjusted. When the angle is increased to 135° the same result is obtained as at 180°: the archentera remain as twins within one ectoderm. The two digestive tracts may point in different directions or the oesophagi may meet and fuse, forming a joint mouth. The skeletons also show that the two partners have adapted themselves to a joint ventro–dorsal polarity. In principle, similar results are attained when two vegetal halves are fused or a vegetal half is added to a whole egg—in both cases with reversed polarity—or a meridional half is combined with a vegetal half. Twins are obtained by fusion of archentera.

A quite different situation, with remarkable consequences, occurs when a vegetal half is transplanted to an animal half, or to another vegetal half, with its polarity reversed in such a way that the micromeres take a central position (Fig. 24(a)$_1$). The reversed part does not directly join in the blastula formation by turning inside out. Instead, both halves segment and curve in their own way, with the result that the one sits like a cap on the other (a)$_2$. Then an opening breaks up under the cap, the new edge fusing with the edge of the cap and establishing a

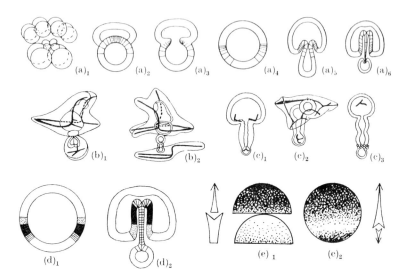

FIG. 24. Diagrams of inversion of the vegetal half. (a)$_1$ The transplantation. (a)$_2$ The animal half sitting as a cap on the vegetal half. (a)$_3$, (a)$_4$
Formation of blastula with the most vegetal material (most densely
hatched) below the equator. (a)$_5$, (a)$_6$ Gastrulation begins with the most
vegetal material (mesenchyme omitted) leaving a vesicle of presumptive
ectoderm (veg$_1$) and a little presumptive endoderm hanging outside the
blastopore (d)$_1$, (d)$_2$. (b)$_1$, (b)$_2$ Two fully differentiated larvae. (e)$_1$ Gradients and polarity at transplantation, (e)$_2$ after reorganization. In
larvae with inverted vegetal half endodermizing action of lithium worked
its way in opposite directions along the two new axes (c)$_1$–(c)$_3$. (From
Hörstadius 1928, 1936b, 1950b.)

blastula (a)$_3$, (a)$_4$. The most vegetal material of the reversed half (hatched) is now situated just under the equator.

Further development of larvae consisting of an animal half with
reversed vegetal half takes the following course (Fig. 24(a)$_5$, (a)$_6$). Both
migration of the primary mesenchyme as well as invagination start
from below the equator, resulting in a kind of gastrula (a)$_6$. The whole
reversed half, however, is not turned into the animal half. A minor
vesicle remains outside the blastopore, connected with the tip of the
archenteron by a narrow string. The vesicle must mainly correspond
to the veg$_1$ of the reversed half, thus presumptive, ectoderm. However, it
apparently contains some veg$_2$-material as well because the vesicle
obtains its own small invagination (b)$_1$, (b)$_2$. The vesicle also attracts
some skeleton-forming cells. Nevertheless the animal half has received

enough endo- and mesoderm to develop as a pluteus. The fact of theoretical interest is that all the mesenchyme and endoderm material according to its polarity ought to have invaded its own veg_1-region, but instead the animal half has had the power to attract the majority of this vegetal material. This larger part differentiates as a pluteus with a small gastrula hanging outside the anus $(b)_1$, $(b)_2$. In animal halves implanted micromeres suppress the animal tendencies to extend the tuft and instead induce ciliated band and stomodaeum formation. In spite of the state of opposition in this case the animal material attracts mesenchyme and archenteron, in a direction actually opposite to its polarity. The large

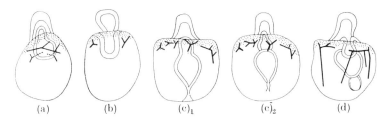

FIG. 25. Strange development of whole larvae animalized by an agent isolated from sea-urchin eggs (see text for explanation).

animal half attracts the greater part, the small veg_1 a correspondingly smaller part. In the light of the strong inductive capacities of vegetal cells, this guiding action of the animal region affords another illustration of animal–vegetal interactions (Hörstadius 1928, p. 74). In the pluteus the presumptive regions of the archenteron have been used in a manner different from the normal—compare Fig. 3(m) and Fig. 18 $(c)_1$, $(c)_2$ with Fig. 24 $(d)_1$, $(d)_2$.

In this connexion it may be appropriate to mention another strange case of animal attraction capacity which, however, is not the result of transplantations. When morphogenetic agents isolated from sea-urchin eggs were tested some were found to act as both animalizing and radializing (see pages 164, 168 and Fig. 55). With one substance whole eggs were transformed into larvae of the type of Fig. 25(a), (b). An expert would probably like to turn them upside down and interpret them as partial exogastrulae. However, with such vegetalization it would be expected that the skeleton and the ciliated band, if any, would be located near the ectodermal pole. The fact that the larva $(c)_1$ and $(c)_2$ was observed and sketched at about a two-hours' interval has made an interpretation possible: the comparatively small archenteron is, in $(c)_1$, so forcefully stretched towards the ectodermal stomodaeum inside the ciliated band that the intestine and ectoderm in the anus region are drawn out to a very thin epithelium; in (c)$_2$, this has ruptured, the whole endoderm being pulled to fuse with the stomodaeum. In (d) another larva in which the intestine has lost the connexion with the ectoderm can be seen. In Fig. 25(a) and (b) the bulge above the band is the animalized ectoderm of the animal pole, and the interior sac is the combined stomodaeum and archenteron.

Another combination with an unexpected reaction involves fusion of two vegetal halves in tandem arrangement, the one on top of the other (Fig. 26(a)$_1$). After passing through a cap stage, with the lower half as the

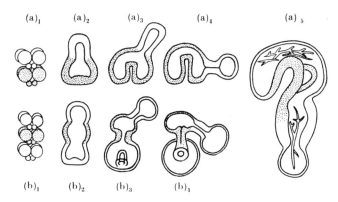

FIG. 26. (a)$_1$–(a)$_5$ When a vegetal half has been transplanted on top of another vegetal half the upper half migrates down along the side of the lower until the endodermal regions make contact with each other. (b)$_1$–(b)$_4$ When three vegetal halves are placed on top of each other the upper half migrates along the side of the middle one which in its turn migrates along the lowest one until endoderm reaches endoderm. (From Hörstadius 1950*a*.)

cap, the upper half sits like a finger-stall on the animal pole of the other (a)$_2$. The lower half begins to gastrulate. The upper half is evidently uneasy in the animal environment; it starts a migration down along the side of the lower partner until the two presumptive endoderm regions meet and partly fuse (a)$_3$–(a)$_5$. The *veg*$_1$ of both differentiate as ectodermal vesicles containing some spicules (a)$_5$ (Hörstadius 1928, 1950*a*). The same trend of fusion of vegetal regions is illustrated by placing three vegetal halves in a series (b)$_1$. The upper half is migrating down along the side of the middle one which simultaneously is moving down towards contact with the endoderm region of the lowest individual (b)$_3$, (b)$_4$.

Although the endoderm regions fused in the experiments with two halves, no united larvae could appear because the angle between the partners was too great after the migration. However, Balinsky (1932) reports a giant harmonious larva after having placed a whole 4-cell stage of *Strongylocentrotus droebachiensis* on top of another.

When an animal half was replaced upside down on its vegetal half, and when two meridional halves were transplanted together with the outside of the one against the inside of the other, the larvae passed through cap stages but gave plutei with only slightly disturbed bilateral symmetry (Hörstadius 1928, p. 70).

Induction versus quantity and distance

Many of the experiments so far described prove that some fragments have a constitution which does not allow an harmonious differentiation. Isolated animal halves, an_1- or an_2-rings, do not gastrulate, and ciliated band and stomodaeum usually fail to appear. Vegetal fragments may form ovoid larvae or exogastrulae instead of plutei. On the other hand, remarkable cases of regulations may be observed. In spite of removal of polar material, an_1, and/or micromeres, typical larvae with tufts and skeletons are obtained. The inductive power of micromeres is spectacular, turning presumptive ectoderm to endoderm, and possibly creating a new axis. The cleavage of the sea-urchin eggs allows manipulations with nearly mathematical exactitude. However, the interpretation of the results cannot often be made in a quantitative way. For a study of regulations along the egg axis, local vital staining as well as count of primary mesenchyme cells are valuable tools.

A vegetal half, containing a little less than a third of the presumptive ectoderm, can in some cases differentiate as a small pluteus (see Fig. 13 (*Pl*)). In order to achieve this harmonious development one is apt to assume ectodermization of presumptive endoderm, and a proportionate reduction of the number of primary mesenchyme cells. Vital staining was performed both with the transplantation and the pipette method. In no case was conversion of presumptive endoderm to ectoderm found. In some larvae the ecto–endoderm dividing line coincided with the veg_1–veg_2 limit. In the majority of the larvae, however, part of the veg_1-cells participated in the invagination. An extreme case is presented in Fig. 27(a). Thus no regulation of the ecto–endoderm limit towards a more harmonious system took place; instead, presumptive ectoderm became endodermized (Hörstadius 1935, p. 302, 1936*b*).

The number of primary mesenchyme cells produced by micromeres does not seem to be much influenced by the constitution of the larvae. Counts in animal halves with implanted 4, 2, or 1 micromeres resulted, in most cases, in the expected number which could be formed by each micromere, normal larvae having about 60 (1935). However, in some larvae the number was lower than expected. A more detailed investigation of the number of cells in larvae of the following composition

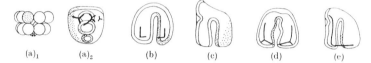

$(a)_1$ $(a)_2$ (b)   (c)   (d)   (e)

FIG. 27. $(a)_1$ Vital staining of a veg_1-blastomere of a vegetal half. $(a)_2$ A part of the presumptive ectoderm has invaginated as endoderm. (b)–(e) After removal of macro- and micromeres such mesomeres were stained which after closure of the cleavage stages would get into contact with the remaining macro- and micromeres. (b), $8+2+2$. (c) $8+2+0$. (d), $8+1+1$. (e), $8+1+0$. In the presence of micromeres endodermized material reaches the tip of the archenteron, (b), (d). (From Hörstadius 1936*b*.)

$8+4+4$ (control), $8+2+2$, $4+2+2$, an_2+4+4, and $0+4+4$ showed that the mean value varied between 58·2 and 61·1. (In larvae with two micromeres the numbers doubled.) It appears from this material that each micromere forms its normal number of primary mesenchyme cells regardless of reduction of animal or vegetal material. The formation of skeleton-forming cells after removal of the micromeres is described on page 60.

When the micromeres were stained before implantation into an animal half it was frequently found that they solely gave rise to mesenchyme, but in some blastulae blue material remained in the wall and was later found at the tip of the archenteron (Hörstadius 1935, p. 331). The latter case explains the reduced number of mesenchyme cells in some larvae, as just mentioned. On the other hand, the total number of cells expected, together with lack of micromere material in the archenteron, prove that the appearance of an induced archenteron is due, not to the participation of implanted material but to an induction, presumably by transmission of some substance between cells (compare Czihak and Hörstadius 1970).

Does veg_2 also have the power to induce endoderm? A glance at Fig. 15(c) and Fig. 22(b), (d), (e) does not give a definite answer; the invagination could be derived from the veg_2-material present. An agar-pipette was used to stain those mesomeres which, after closure of cleavage stages and deprived of macro- and micromeres, would come into contact with the remaining ones. According to Fig. 27(b) and (d), presumptive ectoderm in the combinations $8+2+2$ and $8+1+1$ has been brought to invagination up to the tip of the archenteron, while in $8+2+0$ and $8+1+0$ the endodermized material does not reach so far (c), (e). In connexion with Fig. 22 it was noticed that the process of development is more harmonious when micromeres are present, as these form primary mesenchyme which possesses strong inductive power. We now find that veg_2 is able both to induce (Fig. 27 (c) (e)) and to produce skeleton-forming cells (Fig. 15 (c)) (Hörstadius 1936b).

At first sight some of the reorganization processes do not seem logical when compared to each other. If the micromeres are not counted, the ratio of presumptive ectoderm to presumptive archenteron is about $3:1$ in the egg. When a meridional half is fused with an animal half (see Fig. 17) the volume is normal but the ratio is $7:1$. After removal of two macro- and two micromeres (see Fig. 22) the ratio is $5:1$. Owing to an endodermization, the preponderance of the presumptive ectoderm is equalized. However, when an animal half or the entire presumptive ectoderm is combined with 4 micromeres these small cells are able to induce a harmonious archenteron (see Fig. 15). An isolated veg_2-ring, representing only endoderm material, grows into a larva with both ectoderm and skeleton (see Fig. 16). These examples speak in favour of regulation towards harmony, *sensu* Driesch. However, other experiments show the contrary—for example, animal forces suppressing vegetal tendencies ($8+\frac{1}{2}+0$, Fig. 22(e); an_1+0+1, Fig. 16). In vegetal halves with a ratio of $1:1$ a trend towards harmony should lead to a smaller archenteron, but the development proceeds in the opposite direction (Fig. 27(a)). It is evident that reorganization in an animal or a vegetal direction is a matter of quantity, but it occurs in a complicated manner. A really conspicuous effect is attained only when strong vegetal material borders on presumptive ectoderm, causing a profound change in the gradient system ($8+0+4$, meridional + vegetal half). Changes along the egg axis are less striking. The enormous vegetal preponderance in vegetal halves, $1:1$, leads only to slight endodermization, if any, and the veg_1 can suffice to give ectoderm to a whole pluteus. In other halves, however, the endodermization may be much stronger, leading to an exogastrula with only a small ectodermal vesicle.

A test of the strength of the entire vegetal region in its action along the egg axis against increased animal material was carried out by adding animal halves to the animal end of whole 16-cell stages (1950a). The addition of one animal half, following a cap stage, led to formation of typical gastrulae, the tuft being normal or slightly enlarged. The further development resulted in plutei with too large an oral lobe, and as a rule, also too large a stomodaeum. It is evident from the shape of the plutei that the added animal material was incorporated in the gradient system, but full balance was not achieved. Attempts were made to state whether the ecto–endoderm limit had been exceeded, but without success. The addition of two animal halves gave varying results (Fig. 28). In three of

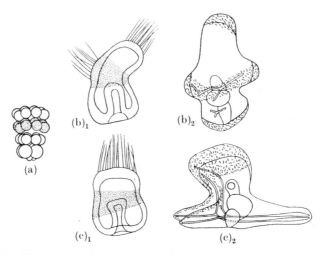

Fig. 28. If two animal halves are added to a whole egg, (a) the animal tuft is more or less extended or also double, $(c)_1$, $(b)_1$. The half next to the egg vitally stained is shown as stippled. A pluteus may develop, although with a considerably enlarged oral lobe, $(c)_2$. In other cases no reorganization to a single gradient system nor to bilateral symmetry has occurred, $(b)_1$, $(b)_2$. (From Hörstadius 1950a.)

the successful cases a reorganization into a single gradient system took place as only one—somewhat enlarged—animal tuft appeared $(c)_1$. A pluteus having an enormously enlarged oral lobe with a large ciliated field is shown in $(c)_2$. The surplus of animal material was too large to allow moulding into a typical form. In $(b)_1$ both the added halves have developed tufts. The absence of a tuft formed by the whole egg below the stained area is, however, a sign of a slight remodelling of the gradients. The fully differentiated larva $(b)_2$ with an animal field and two ciliated bands is of the radial type obtained in many experiments where animalization is produced by chemical means. The digestive tract does not appear to increase in size in order to cope with the large ectoderm, but the contrary

occurs. In this combination the ratio of presumptive ectoderm to presumptive archenteron is 7:1, the same as occurs after fusion of a meridional half with an animal half (see Fig. 17). The difference in regulation
is striking. The reason why harmonious larvae are not obtained after
extension of the egg axis with animal halves seems to be that the added
material is, so to speak, beyond the immediate reach of the vegetal
forces.

One of the first discoveries in experimental embryology was that
plutei develop from meridional half and quarter fragments. On the
other hand, it was not possible to obtain two plutei from one egg after

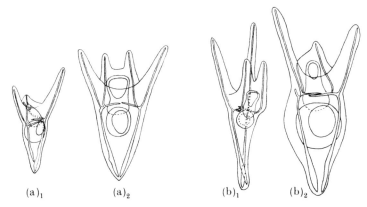

$(a)_1$ $(a)_2$ $(b)_1$ $(b)_2$

FIG. 29. Two plutei cannot be obtained after a transverse section, but
can after two transverse sections if the animal and vegetal fragments
become fused. $(a)_1$, $(a)_2$, $an_1 + 0 + 4$, $an_2 + 4 + 0$. $(b)_1$, $(b)_2$, $8 + 0 + 4$,
$0 + 4 + 0$. (From Hörstadius 1936b.)

transverse section. An animal fragment must contain veg_2-material to
be able to gastrulate, form skeleton and grow to a pluteus. The smallest
vegetal fragments capable of similar development are certain vegetal
halves. Two plutei can, however, be produced if two transverse cuts are
made, the middle fragment left alone and the polar fragments brought
together: $an_1 + 0 + 4$ and $an_2 + 4 + 0$, respectively $8 + 0 + 4$ and $0 + 4 + 0$
(Fig. 29). This provides further support for the double gradient hypothesis. In all the dwarf larvae suitable conditions are present for creating
a properly balanced system.

How far is the nucleus necessary?

Tests have been made to determine whether pieces of the most vegetal
cytoplasm (without nucleus) of a fertilized egg have the same inductive
power as micromeres when implanted in an animal half. No such effect

was found: instead, the experiment revealed extraordinary properties of the blastomeres. By means of the pigment band pieces of vegetal and animal cytoplasm were isolated and were brought into animal halves or $8+veg_1+0$. When micromeres are implanted in this way they stick somewhere to the wall or become incorporated in the wall in the opening of the closing cleavage stage. There is a remarkable reaction against cytoplasm. The blastomeres react to the cytoplasm as to an undesirable intruder, using two methods to get rid of this foreign body. The margins of the open late cleavage stage can bend down towards the piece of cytoplasm, seize it and expel it, as shown in Fig. 30. The blastomeres are

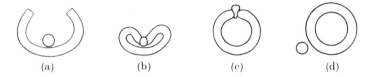

(a)   (b)   (c)   (d)

FIG. 30. (a) A piece of vegetal cytoplasm (without nucleus) of a fertilized egg put into an animal half before it has closed. (b)–(d) The edges of the half-blastula bend down, seize the lump of cytoplasm and eject it. The host can also make an opening between the blastomeres to let the implanted piece fall out. (From Hörstadius 1928.)

also experts in another technique. If the connexion between the cells is rather loose after treatment with Ca-free sea-water, the blastomeres make an opening between themselves large enough to let the implanted piece fall out.

In order to avoid such reactions, the piece of cytoplasm was implanted some two hours after isolation of the animal halves or $8+veg_1+0$ through the smaller opening when they had begun to close. No effect was found after implantation of vegetal cytoplasm as compared to control fragments, or to fragments with implanted animal cytoplasm (Hörstadius 1935, p. 358). Berg and Cheng (1962) tested a possible effect of diffusible substances by rearing whole and half embryos individually in micro–depression slides in the presence of large numbers of segregated micromeres, or macromere–micromere mixtures. However, no animalization or vegetalization was observed.

Many observations have been made concerning the cleavage of enucleated cells (Ziegler 1898; Wilson 1904; and others mentioned in Lorch *et al.* 1953). Asters are formed in spite of the nucleus having been removed, and the cytoplasm may start dividing. This may begin in a fairly normal way but the progressive fragmentation as a rule becomes more and more pathological and the 'cells' incapable of differentiation and participation in the formation of tissue and organs. When 2- and 4-cell blastomeres of sea-urchin eggs were enucleated by micromanipulator (Lorch *et al.* 1953) and such 'cells' became included in the blastocoele, they did not influence the differentiation of the host to pluteus. It is important to state that such dividing cytoplasm is not to be considered as dead. While cytolysing cells have lost the specific permeability characteristic of living cells and quickly become deeply stained by trypan blue, the enucleated and dividing mass remained practically impermeable to trypan blue and was not stained even after two or three days. In another series of experiments the nuclei were removed from either the four animal or the four vegetal blastomeres of 8-cell stages (Hörstadius *et al.* 1953), which were left in contact with the intact halves. The 37 animal halves with attached enucleated vegetal cytoplasm did not reveal any vegetal influence as compared with the control animal halves. However, 8 of the 37 vegetal halves showed a marked animal influence—that is, they formed more or less well-developed plutei, whereas the control larvae never displayed a comparable degree of harmonious differentiation. The result gives the impression that vegetal induction is dependent upon nuclear action while animal influence can be propagated as diffusion from enucleated cytoplasm. As the material was scanty, further investigations are required to support such a tentative conclusion.

Parallelism of morphogenetic and metabolic processes

Child (1936) has described differential reduction of methylene blue and janus green in the early development of sea-urchin and starfish eggs. He describes a reduction gradient in cleavage stages and young blastulae decreasing from the animal towards the vegetal pole (basipetal), and another gradient in the late blastula in the opposite direction (acropetal). A study of reduction gradients in larvae of different constitution has been undertaken (Hörstadius 1952). A weak staining with janus green gives a light greyish-blue colour which at reduction changes into light red; after further reduction the colour vanishes completely. In this way a double check of the reduction process is obtained. About one thousand unstained early cleavage stages were placed in a drop of sea-water enclosed by a vaseline wall. In the centre, which was cleared of eggs, some stained eggs were placed for observation. A coverslip was added and gently pressed down until all air bubbles disappeared. Because of the large number of eggs the oxygen supply became exhausted.

Within an hour or two the reduction phenomena became visible and could be followed individually.

Child's findings have been confirmed. In the early mesenchyme blastula, the change into red starts in the vegetal wall and spreads laterally and vertically (Fig. 31(a)$_1$). When it reaches the neighbourhood of the equator, a new reduction centre appears at the animal pole (a)$_2$. This region too becomes enlarged, and the last region to change colour forms a ring about half-way between the animal pole and the equator (a)$_3$. At this time the second reduction step, the disappearance of the colour, starts at the vegetal end, and the procedure is then repeated (a)$_3$.

In animal halves, with their lack of gastrulation and dominance of animal properties, there is no vegetal reduction centre. Instead, the process starts at the animal pole and continues all round the blastula (b). In vegetal halves the picture is the reverse, as in most cases there is only a vegetal gradient (c). In a few larvae, however, a delayed animal centre was also observed. This is in keeping with the fact that some isolated vegetal halves possess animal qualities in such a large degree that they can form an animal tuft and differentiate as plutei (see Fig. 13).

It is particularly interesting to study the effect of implanted micromeres. When implanted laterally in a whole egg they induce a vegetal centre with archenteron and spicules (see Fig. 19). This induction also includes the formation of a new reduction centre (Fig. 31(d)). When four micromeres are implanted into the vegetal region of an animal half the result is a small pluteus (8+0+4, see Fig. 15). In isolated animal halves the reduction started at the animal pole, and no vegetal gradient ensued. It is seen now that the micromeres change the system to a complete counterpart of that for a normal larva (Fig. 31(e)). The reduction begins in the vegetal wall and spreads upwards; a second animal centre starts later, and the last region to be reduced is at the same level of the larva as in whole eggs (Fig. 31(e)$_4$ and (a)$_3$ respectively).

Since Herbst in 1892 made the remarkable discovery that lithium ions added to sea-water vegetalize sea-urchin eggs many substances have been found to be capable of vegetalizing or animalizing larvae (see Chapter 11). Morphologically, the effect of the agents seems in detail to conform to the results after removing animal or vegetal material, as illustrated in Fig. 32. Accounts are given below of several studies made to determine whether the developmental and physiological characteristics of the morphologically new regions are identical with their counterparts in normal larvae.

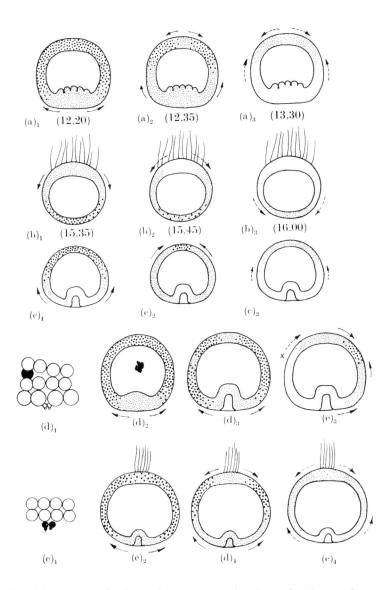

FIG. 31. Change of colour of janus green showing reduction gradients. Large dots, blue; small dots, red; no dots, the colour has faded. Arrows indicate course of reduction, numerals time of observation. (a) Normal late blastula. (b) Animal half. (c) Vegetal half. (d) Micromeres implanted between an_1 and an_2. (e) Micromeres implanted into an animal half. (From Hörstadius 1952.)

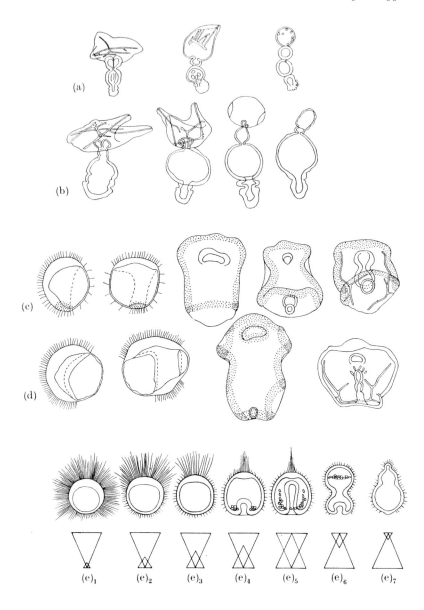

FIG. 32. (a), (b) Embryos of vegetal type (exogastrulae); (a) obtained by reducing the animal material, (b) by lithium ion treatment. (c), (d) Embryos of animal type; (c), obtained by reducing the vegetal material, (d), by animalizing treatment before fertilization. $(e)_1$–$(e)_4$ Different degrees of animalization and $(e)_6$, $(e)_7$ of vegetalization of whole larvae, as well as assumed relations of the gradients. (a)–(d) from Lindahl 1941b, (e) from Gustafson 1965.)

An example of complete correspondence is provided by a further study of reduction gradients in whole embryos animalized or vegetalized by chemical means. As in vegetal halves (Fig. 31(c)) no animal reduction gradient was found in blastulae vegetalized by lithium (Fig. 33(b)). In eggs treated with trypsin the animalization was not complete (Fig. 33(a)). The tuft is considerably enlarged but the larva forms an archenteron, although of much reduced size. In normal eggs the reduction starts at the vegetal pole, the animal centre appearing later. In the trypsin

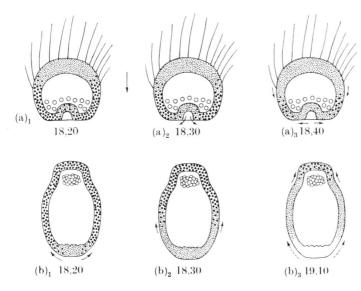

FIG. 33. Reduction gradients illustrated by colour changes of janus green in whole embryos, (a) animalized by trypsin, (b) vegetalized by lithium ions. (From Hörstadius 1955.)

larvae the sequence is reversed, the animal reduction proceeding much faster than the vegetal, the last reduced region lying below the equator, contrary to the animal position in normal eggs.

The biochemical background of the gradients of reduction is not known in detail. According to investigations and reviews of the problem (Bäckström 1961, 1963; Lallier 1964, p. 178) the reduction gradients may be due to differences in the distribution of reducing substances or they may correspond to an unequal distribution of enzymes catalysing oxidation-reduction reactions.

Lithium acts along the vegetal–animal axis. Cleavage stages with reversed vegetal half (see Fig. 24) were transferred to sea-water with

5 per cent isotonic LiCl. Study of a number of larvae showed that the endodermization did not affect the larva as a whole. It was possible to state how the action worked its way along the two axes independently, thus in opposite directions. The veg_1-ectoderm vesicle became strongly diminished; the endoderm gained ground also in the animal half $(c)_1-(c)_3$ Fig. 24. In some cases the veg_1 was completely endodermized and the larva could hardly be distinguished from a typical exogastrula.

The vegetalizing effect of lithium ions has been tested also on animal halves. Such halves of 8-cell stages, following isolation, were placed in sea-water containing LiCl (*Echinocyamus pusillus*, von Ubisch (1925c, 1929). In a certain relation to the strength of the Li-concentration the following types were recorded: larvae with stomodaeum and small archenteron, plutei, gastrulae of vegetal type, and exogastrulae.

The far-reaching parallelism between the action of lithium and that of implanted micromeres provided the impetus to test the vegetalizing power of animal fragments which were themselves vegetalized by Li (Hörstadius 1936b). The eggs used in the experimental series of Fig. 34 were of the animal type, as control animal halves had a much enlarged tuft and developed into ciliated blastulae (b), (c). The an_2-cells of isolated animal halves were lightly stained from contact with agar with Nile blue (a). Thus the vegetal region of the blastulae was recognizable (d). The stained halves were immediately placed in 95 per cent sea-water $+$ 5 per cent isotonic LiCl-solution (d). Some of these halves were allowed to grow to full differentiation to control the Li-action. This was so strong that the animal halves differentiated as ovoid larvae (e). The stained vegetal region of Li-halves were isolated (f) and transplanted to the an_2-side of a normal animal half (g). These halves would have developed as (k), (c) if left alone. The drawings (h)–(j) illustrate the development of one of the larvae with implanted an_2-Li-material. The tuft was only slightly extended (h) and became somewhat diminished (i). The implant was situated like a plug in the vegetal wall, which was not thin as in animal halves (b), (c), (k) but thickened as in a normal late blastula before gastrulation (h). An invagination occurred. The implanted material formed only the tip of the archenteron, the rest being an_2-material which by induction had been transformed to endoderm (i). The final result was a pluteus with typical digestive tract and skeleton (j). Against this proof of Li having converted an_2-material to cells with the same inductive capacity as micromeres, the objection might be made that the action was due to Li left in the implant. This doubt was nullified by taking a piece from the animal pole of Li-blastulae

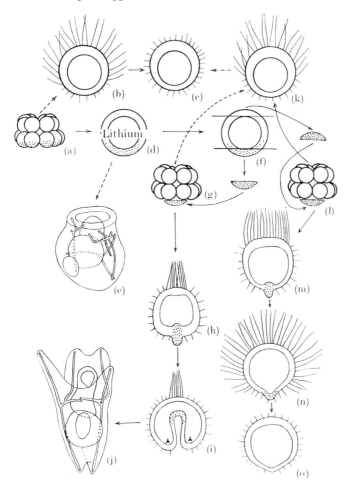

Fig. 34. Development of a pluteus larva from an animal half after implantation of the most vegetal part of another animal half that had been vegetalized by lithium ions. See text for further explanation. (From Hörstadius 1936*b*.)

(f), staining it and adding it to the vegetal side of a normal animal half (l). The further development of this larva continued in the proper animal direction (m), (n), (o).

Another indication of metabolic alterations in larvae of varying animal–vegetal constitution was obtained by counting mitochondria (Lenicque *et al.* 1953). Mitochondria were vitally stained with Nile blue and their distribution along the animal–vegetal axis was studied in late blastula and gastrula stages of whole eggs, animal and vegetal halves,

and animal halves with implanted micromeres. According to Fig. 35(a)
the mitochondrial curve of isolated animal halves differs markedly from
that of vegetal halves. Implantation of micromeres into animal halves
converts the curve into a more vegetal type. The effect is clearly a
function of the number of micromeres implanted. The curve of a control
whole egg lies between those of animal halves with 4 and 8 micromeres.
Similar reactions were reported also after animalization by iodosobenzoic
acid and vegetalization by lithium (Gustafson and Lenique 1952). The
Li-larvae show a more even distribution along the animal–vegetal axis

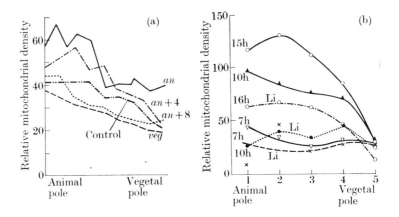

Fig. 35. (a) Distribution of stainable mitochondria along the animal–
vegetal axis in late blastulae–early gastrulae (control), in isolated
animal (*an*) and vegetal (*veg*) halves as well as in animal halves with 4
(*an*+4) or 8 (*an*+8) implanted micromeres. (b) Density of stainable
mitochondria in normal and LiCl-treated blastulae. ((a) from Lenique
et al. 1953, (b) from Gustafson and Lenique 1952.)

than in the controls (Fig. 35(b)). However, these observations do not
illustrate the occurrence of all existing mitochondria. Electron microscope studies in fact indicate a uniform distribution in animal, equatorial,
vegetal, and mesenchyme cells (Berg *et al.* 1962). As various inhibitors
of respiration and oxidative phosphorylation have been found to inhibit
the uptake of stain (Gustafson 1969, p. 194) it is likely that the gradients represent particularly active mitochondria. Another sign of variation of functional capacity is that the maximal density in the span from
10 to 15 hours in normal larvae (Fig. 35(b)) has moved from the animal
pole in a vegetal direction to a level which approximately corresponds
to maximal cytochromoxydase, as shown in Fig. 54(a).

No effect of stratification by centrifugation

Sea-urchin eggs in which the cytoplasm has been stratified by centrifugal force are able not only to develop, but also to differentiate in conformity with the original egg axis. The centrifugal force may act at any angle to the egg axis, and therefore the displaced substances may occupy any position in relation to the polarity of the egg. Nevertheless, normal development ensues (Lyon 1906a, b; Morgan and Lyon 1907; Morgan and Spooner 1909).

Centrifuged sea-urchin eggs have later been subjected to many investigations, particularly by Harvey (1932–51, review 1956). She found, in eggs of the American *Arbacia punctulata* at the light centripetal pole, a cap of oil, then a clear layer containing the egg nucleus, followed by a thin layer of mitochondria, a large region of yolk and, at the centrifugal pole, the dark-reddish pigment. Harvey centrifuged unfertilized eggs or fertilized eggs deprived of membrane hanging in a density gradient of 0·85 mol sucrose and sea-water. By strong centrifugation the hanging eggs become stretched and dumb-bell-shaped and then break across the yolk into two spheres, the 'white halves' containing oil, a clear layer with nucleus, mitochrondria, and part of the yolk; the 'red halves', yolk and pigment. By further centrifugation the white halves can be divided into clear and mitochondria quarters, and the red halves into yolk and pigment quarters. Halves and quarters of unfertilized eggs began to develop after fertilization, the white halves and clear quarters containing the nuclei as diploid merogones, the other fragments being haploid. It is remarkable that parthenogenetically-activated red halves could form a clear cytoplasmic sphere and radiation as amphiasters leading to division into a number of 'cells' without nuclei. This strange development continued to the hatching stage but did not bring about any differentiation. Of the nucleated merogones, some of the white halves, some of the red halves, and some of the clear quarters gave small plutei, but permanent blastulae are also reported. The other three quarters were less capable of differentiation.

In other species the stratification may differ because of the varying size of their mitochrondria and yolk platelets (Harvey 1933; Callan 1949). In *Paracentrotus lividus*, for example, the mitochondria get into the centrifugal pole (the eggs have no interior pigment) (Fig. $36(a)_1$). The superficial red pigment band below the equator remains stable, if centrifugation is not excessively rapid, and can therefore be used as a landmark for orientation (hatched regions).

Experiments were made to test whether stratification at different angles would impair the vegetalizing action of lithium ions (Fig. 36). Eggs were stratified and stretched in sucrose gradient and, with the aid of the pigment band, were isolated in groups according to the effect of the force in the direction of the animal–vegetal axis $(a)_1$, reversed

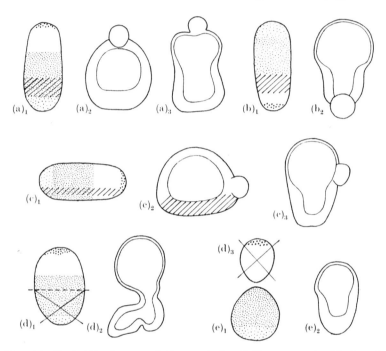

FIG. 36. Unfertilized eggs of *Paracentrotus lividus* were stratified and stretched, and by aid of the remaining pigment band (obliquely hatched) isolated in groups according to effect of the centrifugal force along $(a)_1$, reversed to $(b)_1$, or perpendicular to $(c)_1$ the animal–vegetal axis. The eggs were fertilized and treated with LiCl. The oil cap did not participate in the cleavage, remaining as a lump indicating the light pole. The differentiation as well as the lithium effect followed the egg axis—thus independently of the direction of stratification. Both light (d) and heavy (e) fragments showed strong lithium effect. (From Hörstadius 1953a.)

towards it $(b)_1$, or perpendicular to it $(c)_1$. They were fertilized and reared in a solution of sea-water with 5 per cent isotonic LiCl. Fig. 36(a)–(c) shows larvae in which the oil cap material at the light pole did not participate in the cleavage, but remained as a lump in the wall indicating the centripetal pole. A clear endodermization was obtained in all cases along the vegetal–animal axis of the egg, independently of the atypical distribution of the intracellular inclusions. In (d) a light, and in (e) a heavy half, isolated by glass needle before fertilization, were able to respond to lithium by developing into exogastrulae although containing different substances. The angle to the egg axis was not known.

The development of single fragments from mass cultures of halves and quarters obtained by centrifugation in a sucrose gradient cannot

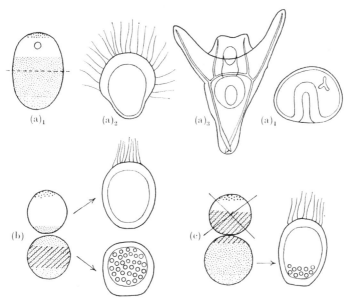

FIG. 37. (a) Stratified unfertilized eggs were divided by a glass needle and fertilized. Larvae were obtained corresponding to animal $(a)_2$, meridional $(a)_3$, and vegetal $(a)_4$ halves. (b) Development of light animal and heavy vegetal half of the same egg to larvae of animal and vegetal type respectively. (c) Heavy animal half with enlarged animal tuft. (From Hörstadius 1953.)

provide adequate information concerning the developing faculty of animal and vegetal halves in the absence of some strata. Stretched eggs were therefore divided by a glass needle equatorially to the centri-fugation axis (Fig. 37$(a)_1$). Plutei, blastulae with enlarged tuft, and gastrulae of vegetal type were obtained, which were derived, apparently, from lateral, animal, and vegetal halves $(a)_3$, $(a)_2$, $(a)_4$. In the larvae (b) and (c) the fragments were identified by the pigment band. In (b) it was visible in the heavy fragment, as the egg was stratified along the animal–vegetal axis. The light animal fragment differentiated as an animal half, and the heavy vegetal fragment in a vegetal direction. In (c) the egg axis was reversed in relation to the stratification. The light pigmented vegetal fragment did not develop. The heavy animal partner produced an enlarged tuft and its vegetal wall showed no sign of gastrulation (under experimental conditions, cells often invade the blastocoele without being true primary mesenchyme cells).

It is an amazing fact that the egg axis remains as the basis for differentiation in spite of stratification deviating at any angle, lithium acting independently of the position of displaced particles, and isolated animal fragments, for example, differentiating in an animal way although containing quite different material: centripetal or centrifugal layers. The stability of the egg axis is often attributed to the cortex which should remain unaffected by the centrifugal force. Another possibility would be the presence of an endoplasmic reticulum as an immovable scaffold.

Determination proceeds in time

In the course of development, the potencies of different regions of the sea-urchin larva become more and more restricted. This progressive determination has been analysed by means of isolations and transplantations at different stages. The early literature provides no reliable information on fragmentations of uncleaved eggs, nor on the stages following early cleavage when isolations were made at random. von Ubisch (1925c, 1931, 1933) isolated animal halves of the elongated blastulae of *Echinocyamus*. These developed into ciliated blastulae— blastulae with band and stomodaeum. As the stage of isolation is not stated, the results do not reveal anything about progressive determination. Jenkinson (1911a) was able to section mesenchyme blastulae and gastrulae at desired levels, and found that fragments of gastrulae had less power of regulation than earlier stages.

The technique with glass needles and local vital staining has facilitated more thorough analysis of the stages from unfertilized eggs to gastrulae (Hörstadius 1928, pp. 9–20, 33–41, 1936a, 1965; Hörstadius and Wolsky 1936). The determination of cleavage was dealt with in Chapter 5. Even before the egg is fertilized we have found a segregation along the egg axis of the same kind as in early cleavage stages (see page 46); isolated animal halves do not gastrulate; most of them show hypertrophy of the tuft and lack ciliated band and stomodaeum. The appearance of the latter organs is ascribed to influences emanating from vegetal sources. The slow advance of this process is followed by isolating animal and

vegetal halves at intervals from 8-cell stages to the beginning of gastrulae. If 4-cell stages are placed for a short while on a Nile blue agar plate,
the animal or vegetal pole stains sufficiently to permit equatorial
sections to be made of the purely spherical blastulae.

A determination in the vegetal direction of animal blastomeres can be
demonstrated during early cleavage within the short space of time from
8-cell to between 32- and 64-cell stages (Fig. 38). The percentage of
halves with large tuft, later ciliated blastulae, decreases in favour of
blastulae with small tuft and richer differentiation. In vegetal halves the
trend is not so conspicuous.

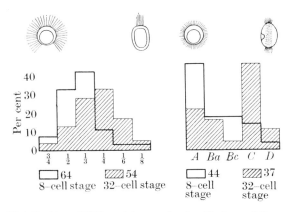

FIG. 38. Distribution of different types of animal halves of *Psammechinus
miliaris* isolated at 8-cell and 32-cell stages respectively. (From
Hörstadius 1965.)

At the top of the diagram in Fig. 39(a) operation stages are depicted
from 16-cell stages about 4 hours after fertilization to the beginning of
gastrulation (16 hours). The late cleavage stages (6 hours) and early
blastulae (8 hours) had to be oriented with the aid of the stained pole.
From late blastulae (10 hours) onwards there is no doubt about the
egg axis. The faculty of extending the tuft is checked at 6–8 hours
(Fig. 39(a)). At 8 hours the normal tuft is formed. The relation between
size of tuft and differentiation into types *A–D* (see Fig. 13) holds also
in the time series (Fig. 39(b)). As to vegetal halves, ovoid larvae were
more numerous after early isolations. The later-isolated halves had a
typical arrangement of the skeleton but more or less lacked the oral lobe
which is normally formed of animal material.

Another method of studying progressive changes is to implant a group

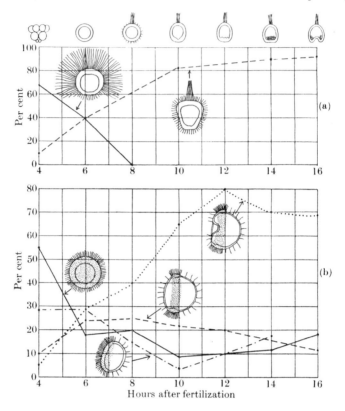

Fig. 39. Isolation of animal halves 4–16 hours after fertilization. The operation stages are indicated above the diagram. (a) Only the extreme types 3/4 and 1/8 of early differentiation are represented. The extension of the animal tuft is inhibited already 8 hours after fertilization, and from this time on the majority of the halves acquire tufts of normal size. (b) The later the isolation is made the less frequent is the most animal type (ciliated blastula), and the more frequent is the type with ciliated band and stomodaeum, that is, the differentiation in accordance with the prospective significance of the material, illustrating the change from a labile gradient system to full determination. (From Lehmann 1945, based on Hörstadius material 1936a.)

of micromeres into animal halves at different times. In the experiment illustrated in Fig. 40, all halves were isolated at 16- or 32-cell stages (4 hours) and the micromeres were implanted at two-hour intervals, beginning immediately after isolation. The drawings below the diagram show how the halves lying isolated before implantation gradually lose the capacity to react to induction from the micromeres. Immediate implantation results, as we know, in plutei, some of them with too small

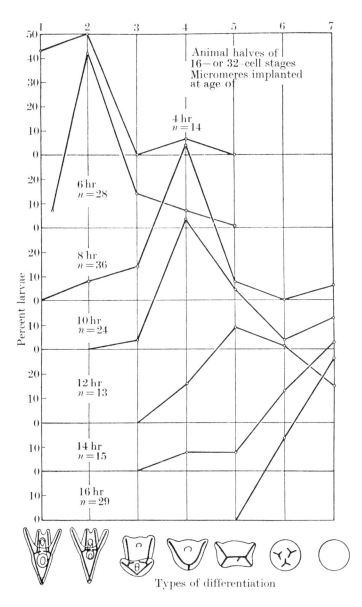

Types of differentiation

FIG. 40. Diagram of types of embryos obtained when animal halves were isolated at 16- or 32-cell stages, and micromeres were implanted at the age of 4–16 hours. n = number of halves. (From Kühn 1955, based on material in Hörstadius 1936a.)

an archenteron. Two hours later the plutei with much reduced digestive tract predominate. At 8 and 10 hours the majority have lost the faculty of forming endoderm. There is no longer any pluteus shape: no arms and only atypical skeleton. After still later implantation stomodaeum fails to appear and the spicules become more irregular. In many blastulae the ectoderm is not even able to entice the micromere descendants into formation of spicules.

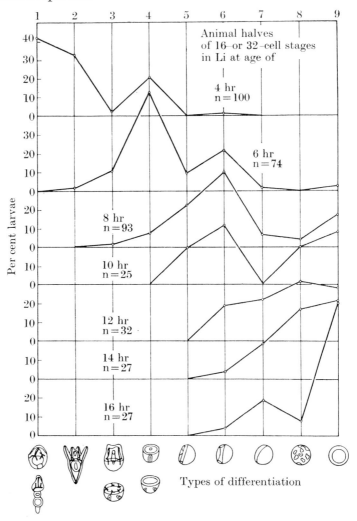

FIG. 41. Distribution of different types of differentiation of animal halves, isolated at 16- or 32-cell stages, and brought into sea-water with 5 per cent isotonic LiCl 4–16 hours after fertilization. (From Kühn 1955, based on material in Hörstadius 1936a.)

In parallel series animal halves were isolated at two-hour intervals, in the stages illustrated in Fig. 39(a), and micromeres were implanted immediately after isolation. The animal halves were then found to be responsive to micromere action at somewhat later stages than in the first series. The animal material evidently restricts its potencies faster in an animal direction when lying isolated than when in contact with its vegetal partner for a longer time.

It has been shown that animal halves may be vegetalized by lithium (see page 78). The drawings below the diagram Fig. 41 show the different types that may be obtained from exogastrulae and ovoid larvae to blastulae. The same kind of experiments as already mentioned were made

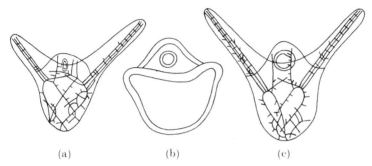

(a)   (b)   (c)

FIG. 42. (a), (c) Plutei of *Echinocyamus pusillus* without digestive tract, obtained from animal halves isolated at 32-cell and 16-cell stages respectively, into which 4 micromeres from the same species had been implanted at a blastula stage. (b) Animal half of the same species, isolated at 32-cell stage and showing mouth and rudiments of anal arms. (From von Ubisch 1933.)

with lithium as agent instead of micromeres. In the first series (see Fig. 41) the halves were all isolated at 16- or 32-cell stages and placed in Li-solution at two-hour intervals. The same gradual decrease in ability to respond to lithium as to the inductive action of micromeres may be observed. In similar experiments when the halves were isolated at different stages, from 4 to 16 hours, and immediately brought into the Li-solution they were more sensitive than those which had been left alone after operation at 4 hours.

The statement that the ectoderm of the animal halves isolated at 16- or 32-cell stages does not react to micromeres implanted at the blastula stage by forming arms with corresponding rods evidently is not valid for all species. Isolated animal halves of the irregular sea-urchin *Echinocyamus pusillus* behave differently by forming traces of arm projections in the absence of micromeres (Fig. 42(b), von Ubisch

1933). After implantation of micromeres in the blastula stage almost complete plutei devoid of digestive tract could appear (a), (c). The animal half at the stage of implantation (not clearly defined) was unable to react to the inductive force of the micromeres by invaginating an archenteron. However, it was still capable of interacting with the primary

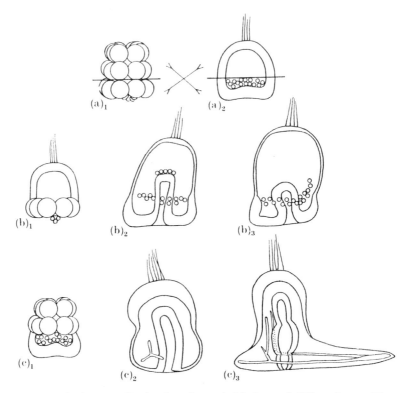

FIG. 43. Exchange of animal and vegetal halves of different age (32-cell stage and beginning gastrula). With an age-difference of 14 hours as in (b) and (c) the difference in differentiation of the components is very pronounced. Both reciprocal combinations could in the end give typical plutei. (From Hörstadius 1950a.)

mesenchyme to form typical anal arms and skeleton pattern with fenestrated anal rods. Only the rods in the body around the non-existent stomach and intestine are irregular.

Animal and vegetal halves of the cleavage stages, blastulae, and incipient gastrulae, with an age difference between the two components varying between 2 and 17 hours, were made to fuse (Hörstadius 1950a). The older blastulae become rather tough, and the needle has to be worked back and forth many times before it cuts through; the edges of each half consequently stick together. This disadvantage was overcome by treating the blastulae with Ca-free sea-water. The treatment must be carefully timed because if it is continued too long the epithelium starts to disintegrate. After successful separation the halves swim about as minute bowls, the vegetal halves with the opening in front, but the edges soon draw closer together and fuse. When a vegetal half is caught and placed against a younger immobile half, no further pressure by a glass ball (see Fig. 9(a)), is necessary as the forward swimming movement of the half-gastrula maintains a steady contact. A greater problem is to keep a swimming animal half from escaping from a young immobile vegetal half.

Reciprocal combinations with age differences of up to 17 hours can in the end produce typical plutei, although the difference in differentiation of the components is very pronounced on the first day after fusion (Fig. 43). An old vegetal half does not, therefore, lose its capacity to inhibit the extension of the animal tuft, or to cause the formation of ciliated band and stomodaeum in the animal material.

7 Determination of the ventro–dorsal axis. Bilateral and radial symmetry

Origin of the ventro–dorsal axis

DRIESCH discovered that complete larvae can arise from isolated blastomeres of 2- and 4-cell stages (see Fig. 1). Boveri (1908) reports four plutei from one egg in some cases. In Fig. 44 four quadruplets are depicted.

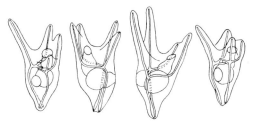

FIG. 44. Four plutei from the isolated quarter-blastomeres of one egg. (From Hörstadius and Wolsky 1936.)

The existence of an animal–vegetal axis even in the mature sea-urchin egg is evident from the appearance of the pigment band in *Paracentrotus*, and from experiments discussed in Chapters 5 and 6. The development of four complete larvae from one egg is evidence against a rigid bilateral organization of the egg in early stages; but there must be a tendency to form a ventro–dorsal axis. The nature of such an organization, and the possibility of its existence before fertilization, or of the ventro–dorsal axis being introduced by the spermatozoon, have been the subjects of many observations and investigations. These, however, have yielded contradictory results and interpretations.

In the holothurians *Cucumaria frondosa* and *Psolus phantapus* a bilateral structure is discernible even in unripe eggs (Runnström and Runnström 1920). These are flattened in the animal–vegetal direction and somewhat stretched perpendicularly to the egg axis. In *Psolus* the axis is heavier at one end. The heavier pole corresponds to the future dorsal, and the lighter to the future ventral side. The eggs of the starfish *Asterina gibbosa* are also rich in yolk. They are spherical or oval. In the latter case, the first furrow is perpendicular to the longitudinal axis. A slight constriction in the 2-cell stage later showed that the furrow separates dorsal from ventral (Hörstadius 1925a).

In normal untreated unfertilized sea-urchin eggs, no morphological traces of bilateral structure have been reported. One way of tackling the problem of an early existing organization has been to study whether even the first cleavage furrow occurs in direct relation to the bilateral symmetry of the larva. However, the question then arose whether such a relation might be inherent in the egg or induced by the sperm (Jenkinson 1911b).

Boveri (1901b, 1902, 1905, 1908), Garbowski (1905), Herbst (1907), Jenkinson (1911b), and Runnström (1914, 1925d) were of the opinion that the first furrow coincides with the plane of symmetry. Driesch (1906, 1908), on the other hand, considered the first cleavage plane to be frontal, but his observation refers to slightly stretched eggs. Boveri (1902) reported that the ventro–dorsal axis can be determined by stretching, as did Lindahl (1932b). von Ubisch (1925a) used local vital staining and came to the conclusion that the first furrow has no fixed relation to the median plane. Contrary to this view, Runnström (1925d) (using a natural mark), as well as Hörstadius (1928) and Foerster and Örström (1933), after vital staining, expressed the view that the first furrow is more often formed in the median and frontal planes than obliquely to those planes. Not convinced of the exactness of the methods hitherto used, Hörstadius and Wolsky (1936) attacked the problem again, using a more refined technique. Small marks of Nile blue made with micropipettes (see Fig. 8) were put near the furrow in the 2-cell stage. The stain soon spread, making a sharp blue boundary towards the other half and yet left the greater part of the first half unstained. The position of the first cleavage plane could be read with great accuracy in the gastrulae and young plutei. Little or no preponderance of the median and frontal planes was found. Decisive proof was obtained by the demonstration that half-larvae isolated in the 2-cell stage correspond to right or left, dorsal or ventral, or oblique meridional parts of the egg (loc. cit.).

There are many incompatible statements on the problem whether sperm induces bilateral symmetry. Selenka (1878), Wilson and Matthews (1895), and Boveri (1901*b*) thought that the entrance of sperm and the position of the first furrow coincide, whereas Garbowski (1905) and Boveri in later observations (see Heffner 1908) came to the opposite conclusion. The problem is technically difficult to tackle. The elevation of the fertilization membrane starts at the site of entry of the sperm but usually the elevation proceeds too fast to allow utilization of this point. Runnström (1925*d*) found 12 eggs in which the membrane only formed a vesicle where the sperm had entered. In all 12 cases the first furrow was lying below this vesicle. The reason for this may perhaps be sought in a certain tension exerted by the membrane rudiment. Hörstadius (1928) stained the side opposite the site of entry in a batch with slow membrane elevation. This point was found in any position in relation to the first furrow. As this furrow is independent of the future ventro–dorsal axis, the assay tells us nothing about the possible effect of the spermatozoa.

Runnström has recently dealt with the problem in two papers. Partial cortical activation was studied (1959) by interrupting the activating impulse by a temporary exposure of the eggs to 32°C, using the method of Allen and Hagström (1955), at different intervals after fertilization. The activated region around the sperm entry is termed proximal, and the opposite side, distal. The site of sperm penetration could sometimes be recognized by a slight membrane elevation, or by a protrusion of the egg surface. In a majority of cases the partially elevated membrane was found to have an equatorial or subequatorial extension which indicates that the spermatozoon enters mainly in these regions. Furthermore, a bulge often appeared on the distal side, thus antipodal to sperm entry. Later, it was often found again in the dorsal lip of the blastopore (no numbers given). These observations led the author to the tentative conclusion that the equatorial and subequatorial ventral region of the egg is more receptive to the spermatozoon than are other regions. Runnström's second paper (1962) describes how eggs were fertilized in the presence of ribonuclease, and showed a pronounced proximal–distal polarity with the axis perpendicular to the animal–vegetal axis which could be recognized by a concavity or flattening of the egg surface. The site of sperm entry was characterized by a small cone-like structure. In treated eggs the great majority of sperm entered the distal-dorsal side of the egg, while in control eggs the result was exactly the opposite. Whereas the first paper showed that sperm entries occurred mainly in the vegetal half, the tables now suggest an equal number in both animal and vegetal halves in the controls and a greater number in animal halves in the treated eggs. Formerly the sperm was supposed frequently to have a determining effect on bilateral organization: these new experiments suggested the opposite interpretation—namely, that a certain degree of organization by the egg influences the site of fertilization. However, further investigations are required to solve this problem.

Treatment of eggs with several substances has brought about changes in shape which are interpreted as signs of an early ventro–dorsal structure. Alkaline sea-water, certain amino acids, and SH-compounds cause the formation of concavities in unfertilized eggs of *Echinocardium cordatum* (Gustafson 1945, 1952). There are two reasons why it is possible, although not proved, that these concavities are expressions of a ventro–dorsal organization before fertilization: their appearance is checked by agents—for example, detergents—which give rise to radial symmetry, and they seem to correspond to concavities which are evoked in fertilized eggs by KCN, or CO in the dark, the most distinct of which, after staining, have been shown to represent the ventral side (Foerster and Örström 1933). Markman (1963) interprets a precocious appearance of ventro–dorsal differentiation brought about by the exposure of fertilized eggs to antibiotics as an indication of ventro–dorsal structure before fertilization. Investigations on similar lines by Runnström (1959, 1962) have already been cited.

Decisive arguments for the existence of two systems of polar organization even in the unfertilized egg are as follows. Eggs brought to development by artificial parthenogenesis differentiate into plutei (Loeb 1899). When meridional halves of unfertilized eggs are fertilized, both halves develop from one egg, the one being diploid and the other haploid. Independently of this difference, pairs could be interpreted as belonging to the left–right, or ventro–dorsal, parts of the egg (Hörstadius and Wolsky 1936). There seems to be no doubt as to the existence of a ventro–dorsal axis in the unfertilized sea-urchin egg. However, this axis is labile. As already mentioned, it is sensitive to stretching. The bilateral symmetry can also be changed by centrifugation before fertilization (Runnström 1925d, Lindahl 1932c, Pease 1939). Runnström states that the pole containing large lipoid granules differentiates into the ventral side. On the other hand, Motomura (1948) found that the centripetal pole became the vegetal pole—if the centrifugal force had caused a movement of the cortical cytoplasm.

The instability of the ventro–dorsal axis is also illustrated by the

development of larvae with radial instead of bilateral symmetry following treatment with certain substances (see page 107). Pease (1941,
1942*a, b*) found after local application of metabolism-inhibiting substances that the inhibited part of the egg produced the dorsal side. The
ventral side in the course of development has higher energy requirements
and is characterized by a maximum of cytochromoxydase activity
(Czihak 1961).

Bilateral organization in fragments and giants

A more thorough study should be undertaken as to how the ventro–
dorsal axis and the bilateral symmetry develop in meridional halves in
comparison with the organization of the egg. Boveri (in Heffner 1908)
thought that the ventro–dorsal axis in halves would rotate through 90°.
Driesch (1908) considered that the axis was reversed in ventral halves
but remained in dorsal halves. Runnström (1914), on the other hand,
was of the opinion that the axis does not change in isolated half-blastomeres.

Hörstadius pointed out in 1928 that the only reliable method to study
whether a stable or a labile bilaterality exists in the early stages would
be to isolate fragments and vitally stain the cut side. In many pairs of
meridional halves of 16-cell stages stained accordingly (Hörstadius and
Wolsky 1936), the development was more or less delayed regarding
skeleton and arms on the left side of the one, and on the right side of the
other, half. As these sides were stained and therefore represented the cut
sides, the halves must be designated as presumptive left and right halves
of the egg (Fig. 45(a)–(c)). However, in other pairs both larvae were
stained in their dorsal parts (Fig. 46(b)$_1$, (b)$_2$). In such cases the one was
clearly ahead of the other in forming the ventral side (b)$_1$, (c)$_1$. No doubt
this was the presumptive ventral part of the egg which differentiated in
the same way as it should have done in the larvae. Its ventro–dorsal
polarity has not changed (b)$_1$, (c)$_1$, (d). However, in the other half the
ventro–dorsal axis was reversed (b)$_2$, (c)$_2$, (d). The adjustment to the
reversal took some time and the differentiation was delayed. The reason
may also be that the material in the presumptive dorsal side had not the
same capacity for ventral differentiation. In pairs from eggs with the
first furrow standing obliquely to the median plane, the results were
variable.

The objection to the interpretation of these results could be raised
that the vital stain has impaired the cut sides, resulting in delayed development of the skeleton in left and right halves, and has turned the stained

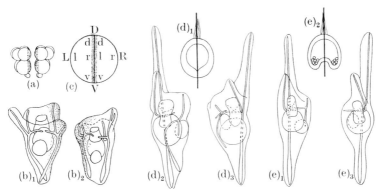

FIG. 45. (a) Meridional halves of a 16-cell stage vitally stained on the cut sides. (b)$_1$, (b)$_2$ A pair of early plutei with stain and delayed development on the cut sides. (c) Diagram of position of the ventro–dorsal axis in a whole egg (capital letters) and in the left and right halves (lower case letters). (d) Skeleton and arms lagging still more behind in left and right halves isolated at blastula stage. (e) After isolation at stage of gastrulation the halves have differentiated as left and right halves of a pluteus. (From Hörstadius 1936a; Hörstadius and Wolsky 1936.)

region of ventral and dorsal halves into a dorsal side. It is known that excessive staining can lead to formation of a dorsal side—see the following paragraph and compare also the inhibition experiments of Pease mentioned on page 96. However, the outcome of the many experiments referred to in this book, in text and figures with stained cell layers or single cells, should show that moderate staining has no injurious effect.

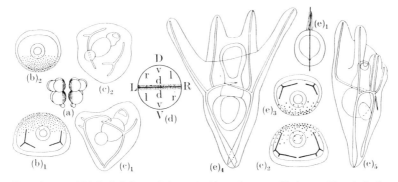

FIG. 46. (a) Vital staining of the cut sides of a 16-cell stage. The stain in the ventral, (b)$_1$, and dorsal, (b)$_2$, half at gastrula stage. (c)$_1$, (c)$_2$ The same halves at a later stage. (d) Diagram showing the inversion of the ventro–dorsal axis in the dorsal half. (e) Similar inversion after isolation at blastula stage. Note the broad ventral side in the ventral half compared to the new narrow ventral side in the dorsal half. (From Hörstadius 1936a; Hörstadius and Wolsky 1936.)

Decisive arguments in the present case are constituted by the following experiments. Isolated meridional halves of 2-cell stages cannot be stained properly as the cut side cannot later be identified with certainty. Studies were made of the development of a great number of unstained half-blastomeres isolated and reared in pairs. Larvae interpreted as left–right and ventral–dorsal pairs were found with about the same frequency as in series with stained halves of 16-cell stages. Furthermore, unfertilized eggs were divided into meridional halves with the pigment band as orientation mark. The halves were fertilized and reared in pairs. The haploid half was smaller and slower in development than the diploid twin. In spite of this difference several pairs were identified as left and right halves. A dorsal half with large nuclei developed because of the diploid state, in spite of the reversal process, somewhat faster than the haploid ventral partner.

The reversal of the axis in the dorsal half (Fig. 46(d)) can be explained in terms of the idea expressed by Lindahl (1932*b*, 1936*a*) in connexion with stretching experiments. Lindahl sucked eggs into a fine pipette and then stained the posterior end of the eggs. This became ventral, provided the staining was moderate. With too intense staining it became dorsal. In some cases, Lindahl obtained larvae with two ventral sides, at the ends of the stretched eggs (Fig. 47(a), (b)). This implies a reversal of

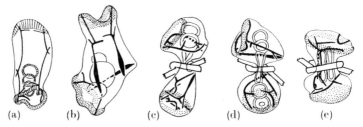

FIG. 47. Biventral larvae were obtained when eggs were stretched (a), (b) or constricted in a meridional plane (c)–(e). (a), (b) from Lindahl 1932*b*; (c)–(e) from Hörstadius 1938.)

the ventro–dorsal axis in a part of the egg in relation to the remainder, as in the separated dorsal halves. Quarter-larvae give plutei as shown in Fig. 44. All meridional parts therefore have the faculty of producing a ventral side. Lindahl now assumes on the presumptive ventral side a centre which inhibits the formation of a similar centre on the opposite side. The results on stretched eggs were confirmed by constriction experiments (c)–(e) (Hörstadius 1938). With slight meridional constrictions only one ventral side is obtained. When the eggs are more tightly constricted, the ventro–dorsal axis may be reversed in the dorsal partner, as in isolated dorsal halves (c)–(e). In stretched and constricted eggs, as well as in isolated dorsal halves, it is consequently the material most distant from the ventral centre which is least inhibited and therefore able to initiate a new ventral side.

The development of isolated blastomeres of 4-cell stages suggests a similar explanation of the rearrangement of bilateral symmetry. Each of the four blastomeres was reared in a separate dish in their circular order in the egg. In some cases two were found to differentiate faster than the other two with regard to the ventral side. These must have

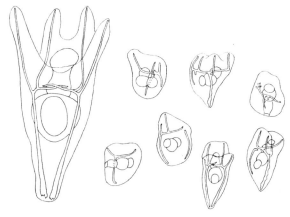

Fig. 48. Control pluteus and seven 1/8-larvae from one egg. (From Hörstadius and Wolsky 1936.)

corresponded to two ventral and two dorsal regions. Other quartets presented one larva much ahead, two intermediate, and one still more delayed in differentiation, no doubt representing one ventral, two lateral, and one dorsal blastomere. In some quartets, however, the results were variable (Hörstadius and Wolsky 1936). Nor did the isolation of one group of 1/8-larvae in circular order give clear evidence of bilateral organization (Fig. 48).

The gradual course of determination of bilateral symmetry was followed by isolating meridional halves from 16-cell stages to blastulae at the beginning of gastrulation (Hörstadius 1936a). Left and right halves of early cleavage stages (4 hours after fertilization) are able to develop into plutei although the skeleton and arms of the cut sides are somewhat delayed (see Fig. 45(b)). In halves isolated 10 hours after fertilization the contrast between sides in each larva is spectacular

(Fig. 45(d)). The originally lateral regions have each produced one perfect pluteus skeleton and well-developed arms and apex, while the cut sides show rudimentary spicules and lack arms. The differences between halves of incipient gastrulae are still greater (Fig. 45(e)). They create the impression of a pluteus divided by a median cut.

The development of ventral and dorsal halves from larvae of different age is of particular interest as it illustrates the changing balance between two opposite ventral centres. The ventro–dorsal axis is completely reversed in dorsal halves isolated 4 hours after fertilization (Fig. 46(a)–(d)). Isolations at about 10 hours can in some cases lead to the same result (e). The ventro-dorsal axis is reversed in the dorsal half and the secondary character of the new ventral side is obvious from its narrowness (e)$_5$ as compared to the typical appearance of the ventral partner.

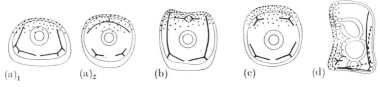

(a)$_1$ (a)$_2$ (b)   (c)   (d)

FIG. 49. After isolation as late as 10–12 hours after fertilization, the dorsal halves may show attempts at forming a ventral side both at the presumptive dorsal and the cut, presumptively most ventral side. (a)$_1$, (a)$_2$ Ventral and dorsal half of the same egg. (b)–(d) Dorsal halves. (From Hörstadius 1936a.)

In other pairs, however, there is a reversal with complications. In the dorsal halves (Fig. 49(a)$_2$, (b)) a new ventral side is formed, to be sure, but on the cut side are found supernumerary spicules, an indication of a tendency to ventrality in the presumptive most ventral region. In (c) and (d) the struggle has ended with a draw. The presumptive dorsal side has managed to develop the largest pair of spicules, and in (d) is seen with the rods growing out in typical pluteus shape, but the ectoderm is thin. Contrary to this, the opposite side has only two small triradiate spicules, but instead the ectoderm forms a thick oral side which in (d) even possesses a stomodaeum. At the beginning of gastrulation (16 hours) there is no sign of reversal, the halves differentiating exactly as dorsal and ventral halves of a pluteus (Hörstadius 1936a, Fig. 6).

The gradual progress of determination of the ventral side has also been established by the application of detergents at different stages (Gustafson and Sävhagen 1949). As the experiments were made with larvae of *Psammechinus miliaris*, the time scale is not quite comparable to that of the fragmentation series with *Paracentrotus* embryos. Up to 6 hours after fertilization the development of a ventral side was checked by the detergents that is, the larvae became radial. From 9 hours onwards no effect was detectable. Between 6 and 9 hours intermediate stages were obtained, as the detergent gradually lost its effect.

A number of transplantation experiments have shed further light on the progress of bilateral determination.

Animal and vegetal fragments of the same age were rotated in relation to each other. A meridional side of 8-cell stages was vitally stained. At the following stage, animal and vegetal halves were isolated and the one partner was transplanted back to the other after rotation through $90°-180°$. Typical plutei appeared when the blastula was round. A complete regulation had taken place. However, when the larvae became elongated, irregularities were observed. Because of faulty fusion the contact had evidently been too narrow to allow of complete interactions. After rotation between presumptive ectoderm and endoderm, $8+veg_1$ and veg_2+4 respectively, the latter seemed to adjust to the ectoderm (Hörstadius and Wolsky 1936).

Animal and vegetal halves of different ages were also brought together (see Fig. 43). Reciprocal combinations with age differences up to 17 hours can, in the end, give typical plutei (see page 90). The transplantations were, of course, made at random regarding the presumptive ventro–dorsal axes. It is striking that the bilateral organization of larvae with age differences varying from only 2 to 8 hours was completely typical (plutei) whereas important aberrations occurred in the larvae with between 14 and 17 hours of age difference. The ciliated bands appeared earlier in the older part, and the bands from the two partners then differentiated independently and were not co-ordinated to a single band. The skeleton was irregularly arranged, and in many cases showed a tendency to radial symmetry. In some larvae the animal and vegetal halves differentiated each according to its own bilateral symmetry, the halves being more or less rotated in relation to each other. Isolated animal and vegetal halves of early cleavage stages are known often to differentiate into larvae with a marked although not always typical, bilateral shape (see Fig. 13). Their bilateral organization at the stage of early isolation is, however, so labile that a reorganization to a unit is possible between young halves of different ages (2–8 hours). The determination evidently proceeded to a considerable extent in the late blastulae and the beginning gastrulae. Only a few perfect plutei were obtained with age differences between 14 and 17 hours (reciprocal

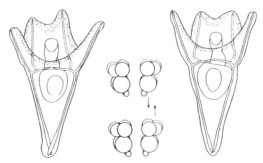

FIG. 50. A pair of typical plutei obtained after exchange of meridional halves between two eggs. (From Hörstadius 1957.)

combinations). It may be assumed that in these larvae the ventro–dorsal axes happened to coincide at the transplantation (Hörstadius 1950).

Meridional halves of 16- or 32-cell stages were exchanged between two eggs (Fig. 50). In all forty-two cases with perfect transplantation both partners in the pair developed into plutei with typical bilateral symmetry. Diagrams of eggs with supposed dominating ventral centre (black) decreasing in the dorsal direction are shown in Fig. 51(a)–(c).

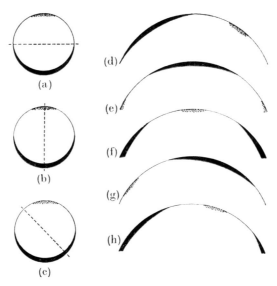

FIG. 51. Diagrams of eggs with a supposed dominating ventral centre (black) decreasing in a dorsal direction. The least inhibited material (dotted area) will be found at the presumptive dorsal pole. (a)–(c), constitution of dorsal and ventral, left and right, and oblique halves. (d)–(h), constitution of flattened whole cleavage stages cut open along radii corresponding to the broken lines in (a)–(c). (From Hörstadius 1957.)

The opposite, least-inhibited material is dotted. The forty-two pairs may be assumed to form all the combinations of halves with the constituents shown in the figures. Regardless of the size of the parts of the ventral centre which come together, complete regulation has always been possible, one side taking the lead and suppressing the other rudiments.

What kind of regulation is possible when two whole eggs are fused into a giant? Several investigators have described the fusion of sea-urchin eggs but have dealt only with random orientation as regards their axes (Driesch 1900*b*, 1910; Garbowski 1904; Janssens 1904; Bierens de Haan 1913*a*, *b*; Goldforb 1914, 1917; Herbst 1926—among others). To study this problem satisfactorily it is imperative to obtain giant larvae with a common animal–vegetal axis. Such giants will have a double number

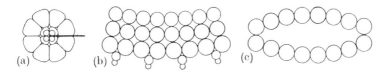

FIG. 52. Fusion of two 32-cell stages to form a giant larva with unitary animal–vegetal axis. (a) The egg is placed on its animal pole and cut along a meridian from the vegetal to the animal pole (heavy line). (b) The 32-cell stage flattened as one layer. (c) A flattened egg placed on top of another, as seen from their animal ends. (From Hörstadius 1957.)

of cells of normal size. In our investigation 32-cell stages were opened with a meridional cut from the centre between the micromeres (Fig. 52(a)). The 32-cell stage was then unrolled and flattened out as in (b). Two such sheets were brought together with their egg axes parallel and with the same polarity under pressure from a piece of a glass capillary tube. The giant blastula formed as a result of this transplantation had a comparatively short egg axis of normal length, but the circumference was twice as large as that of a normal egg. Because of the flattening of the two eggs, the vegetal material was not concentrated in one point but was somewhat elongated. Therefore it was possible that the invagination started at two points but shortly thereafter the two tubes fused at the base, so that the intestine in all cases, and the stomach in most cases, were unitary whereas the first-invaginated parts, the oesophagi, in many cases were double. Several of the giants differentiated as perfect plutei (Fig. 53(a)). Many of them were of pluteus shape but with a supernumerary large spicule in the apex, and sometimes also with an extra piece of ciliated band (c)–(e). These additional structures which represent an attempt to form a second ventral side are thus found in the most distant dorsal part of the larva. The extreme example of doubling is illustrated in (f). It is still a giant pluteus body, with one intestine and stomach but with the other organs duplicated. There are two oesophagi with two mouths facing in opposite directions; two complete ciliated bands (oral fields); and two pairs of skeletons, back to back. The larva has obviously formed two ventral sides as far as possible from each other in the gastrula. The flattened whole cleavage stages may have had the constitution shown in Fig. 51(d)–(h) when cut open along radii corresponding to dotted lines in (a)–(c). Reorganizations within these new heterogeneous systems could lead to the formation of one completely dominating (Fig. 53(a)) or two equal opposite centres (f), or two centres of different strength (c)–(e) (Hörstadius 1957).

Morgan (1895c) and Driesch (1898a, 1900a) paid attention to the problem of number and size of cells in fragments differentiating as plutei. They found that the size is the same as in normal larvae but the number is reduced in direct relation to the size of the fragment. This rule of constant cell size and variable number of cells (Driesch) is valid also when comparing eggs of different size in the same species, the individuals from larger eggs having more, but not larger, cells. The cells during cleavage decrease in size. Boveri (1905) drew attention to the fact that the rule of fixed cell size holds only when the eggs have the same amount of nuclear material. Parthenogenetic eggs develop nuclei of half-size but with double the number of cells; fertilized eggs starting with a monaster have nuclei and cells of double size but only half as many as normal larvae. Decisive for the cell size at the end of cleavage is, therefore, the rule of a fixed nucleus/cytoplasm relationship (Morgan 1895c; R. Hertwig 1903).

The giants illustrated in Fig. 53, which are artificially produced by fusion of cleavage stages, contain a double number of cells of normal size. Genuine giants are those emanating from eggs which, in the ovary, have reached double size of both cytoplasm and nucleus, the larvae consequently consisting of a normal number of cells of double size. Such giant eggs have been found in batches of several species (literature already cited). Many of these eggs did not show normal development. Some of them had evidently arisen from the fusion of two eggs in the ovary, as they had two nuclei. However, both Bierens de Haan (1913c) and Herbst (1926) reported several cases of development into giant plutei with cells of double size. The manner of origin of the giant eggs could not be established. Boveri (1914) has suggested another origin than fusion of two eggs. Instead of a diaster at the last division of oogonia there should appear a monaster giving oocytes with nuclei of double size and the cytoplasm should grow until the normal nucleus/cytoplasm relation has been reached.

In a batch of *Paracentrotus lividus* a great many giant eggs were found. They developed by way of a typical cleavage into giant plutei

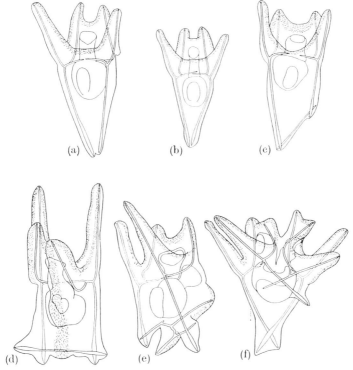

FIG. 53. (a) Giant pluteus. (b) Control pluteus. (c)–(e) Plutei with rudiments of ventral differentiations at their most dorsal end, the apex. (f) Siamese twin with two pairs of skeleton, two oral fields, two mouths and oesophagi. (From Hörstadius 1957.)

with cells of double size (Hörstadius 1971). Some of the larvae, however, deviated from the normal pattern by having one or two supernumerary spicules in the dorsal region of the gastrula. Such pieces of skeleton were still found in some of the plutei, and were reminiscent of similar spicules in the larvae (Fig. 53(c)–(e)). In the latter cases the irregularities were referred to a second ventral centre established in giants with an enlarged equatorial circumference because of which the dominating centre could not completely suppress the opposite rudiment. It is re-markable that the same lack of complete inhibition appears in these larvae which are harmonious in all other respects.

In conclusion, it may be stated that even the unfertilized egg of several echinoderms has a bilateral structure. In eggs of two holothurians and one starfish a ventro–dorsal axis is morphologically established. In sea-urchins the existence of two axes may be traced—for example, from the facts that bilateral larvae derive from artificially activated eggs and that meridional halves of eggs divided before fertilization may differentiate as right–left or ventro–dorsal twins. However, this bilateral

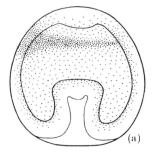 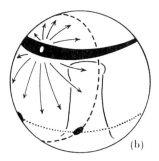

FIG. 54. Diagrams of oral field gradient in an early gastrula. (a) Density of dots combined from by janus-green-stained mitochondria (cytochrome oxidase gradient) and cytoplasm protein staining with azure B. (b) The oral field gradient black, centre white, from which the determination is spreading. The ciliary band develops on the border line (dashes), and the triradiate spicules are formed where this line crosses the circle of primary mesenchyme cells (dotted). (From Czihak 1961, 1962.)

organization is very unstable as the dorso–ventral axis is reversed in dorsal halves. By isolation and transplantation experiments it has been possible to follow how ventro–dorsal determination gradually became established.

Czihak (1961, 1962, 1963) has described a new gradient in sea-urchin development, the oral field gradient. Mitochondria stainable with janus green B were found in denser concentration in the prospective oral field than elsewhere, an indication of a high cytochromoxydase activity. DNA and proteins were stained with azure B and showed a similar gradient in both blastulae and gastrulae. A diagram of the results is shown in Fig. 54. The question may be raised whether this gradient is new. As has been shown several substances changed the shape of un-cleaved eggs in a way interpreted as a sign of a ventro–dorsal structure.

Isolations proved the existence of such an axis in early cleavage stages. The oral gradient may therefore be a late expression of this gradient which Czihak was the first to visualize.

Effect of external agents

Herbst found in 1893 that a weak treatment with lithium could inhibit bilateral symmetry, the larvae instead attaining a radial organization. The use of sea-water without sulphate or the addition of butyric sodium or change of concentration of Na-, K-, Ca-, or Mg-chloride led to the same result (Herbst 1904; Fischel 1909). Since that time a number of substances have been reported as radializing agents.

As there has been some confusion in the interpretation of the relation of bilateral to radial symmetry, a series obtained of intermediate stages from pluteus to radial larva which showed varying sensitivity to 8-chloroxanthine is reproduced in Fig. $55(b)_1–(b)_7$. The transition from bilateral (see Fig. 3) to radial organization is characterized by a straight digestive tract with the mouth in the animal instead of the ventral position. The oral arms and rods decrease in size, first the ventrally-directed parts, and then the parts parallel to the egg axis. The skeleton is then mainly confined to the original skeleton-forming plane where the long anal and body-rods become shorter and the whole pattern irregular, with the appearance of new spicules. In many cases a number of separate skeletal pieces in a ring (d)–(h) are found instead of the normal two. Their triradiate origin is often maintained, with one rod possibly growing very long, but now in the vegetal or animal direction (e), (f), (h). Simultaneously, the ciliated band undergoes a radical transformation. After reduction of the oral lobe it divides into two separate bands perpendicular to the egg axis, one animal round the mouth and one vegetal at the level of the ring of spicules $(b)_7$, (d)–(h). Larvae with radial symmetry may have only one coelomic vesicle which may form a ring around the oesophagus (f) (Czihak 1962).

It is striking that many radializing substances also have an animalizing or vegetalizing effect. The problem is whether this question should not be regarded from the opposite angle and radial symmetry taken to be a consequence of dislocation of the balance in an animal or vegetal direction. In Fig. 55 the larvae (b) and (c) had been treated with 8-chloroxanthine, and (g) and (h) with an endogenous substance respectively, both of which animalize isolated halves, while (d) had been influenced by vegetalizing β-phenyllactic acid and (f) by lithium.

With local ultra-violet radiation Czihak (1962) destroyed the vegetal–

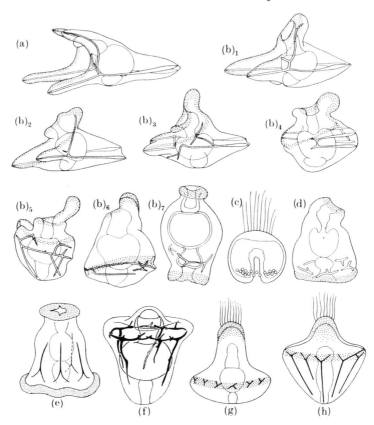

FIG. 55. (a) Normal pluteus. $(b)_1$–$(b)_7$ Larvae treated with 8-chloroxan-
thine showing different degrees of change from bilateral to radial symmetry. (c) The same agent has caused animalization of a gastrula. Radial
symmetry after treatment with 4-phenyllactic acid (d), the detergent Na-
laurylsulphate (e), LiCl (f), endogenous substances (g), (h). Note the coelom
as ring round the oesophagus in *f*. ((a)–(d) from Hörstadius and Gustafson
1954, (e) from Gustafson and Sävhagen 1945, (f) from Czihak 1962,
(g), (h) from Josefsson and Hörstadius 1969.)

ventral corners of the ectoderm of early gastrulae. In spite of destruction
of such crucial points the bilateral symmetry was not affected. However,
after the animal ectoderm had been killed the larvae became radialized,
another result pointing to the importance of an harmonious animal–
vegetal balance for normal development of bilateral symmetry.

Schleip (1929) and Runnström (1931) have advanced the hypothesis
that the bilateral organization could be due to an oblique position of
the vegetal gradient, with its most vegetal point slightly displaced to the

ventral side. Lindahl (1936) assumed that animal and vegetal substances are equally formed on all sides around the pole, but that they diffuse faster on the ventral than on the dorsal side. He also ascribes an organizing capacity to the oral field on the ventral side. A number of isolation and transplantation experiments (Hörstadius and Wolsky 1936) did not confirm the hypothesis of stronger vegetal properties on the ventral side, nor is it compatible with the reversal of the ventro–dorsal axis in isolated dorsal halves.

Sugars occupy a special position as regards both effect on the ventro–dorsal organization and duration of action (Hörstadius 1959, 1960). Eggs of *Psammechinus miliaris* during different periods after fertilization were placed in sugar solutions of different concentrations, the highest consisting of equal parts of isotonic sugar solution and sea-water. The sugar effect was produced not only with the hexose monosaccharides glucose, fructose, galactose, and mannose, but also with the disaccharides sucrose and lactose, as well as with the pentoses xylose and arabinose. A test with ribose proved negative. In weaker concentrations, plutei have a broad and thick oral lobe devoid of oral arms but covered with a large ciliated field (Fig. 56(a), (b)). A stronger action of sugar leads first to an increase of the animal tuft and then to an excessive development of the acron and ciliated band and also of the stomodaeum—the oral field—at the cost of the aboral side, the apex with the body-rods (c), (d). The strongest effect often gives the impression of radialized larvae, but in fact these are probably bilateral larvae (although the skeleton may show radial symmetry) constituted like larvae (e) and (f): the enormous oral field has forced aside the aboral body-wall to a small area round the anus, the lateral parts of the ciliated band having fused in the dorsal midline.

Li-ions intervene in the determination process only during cleavage and early blastula stages (Lindahl 1936) (see interrupted line in the schematic Fig. 56(o)). Animalization can be obtained by using iodosobenzoic acid during the same period (Runnström and Kriszat 1952*b*), by rhodanid ions before fertilization (Lindahl 1936), and by 8-chloroxanthine both before and after fertilization (Hörstadius and Gustafson 1954) (see thin line in Fig. 56(o)). In comparison, the period of sensitivity to sugar does not occur until the time of hatching (see heavy line)—that is, when the sensitivity to vegetalizing or animalizing substances is waning. This indicates that the possibility of interfering with the determination ceases to exist at an earlier stage along the animal–vegetal axis than along the ventro–dorsal axis.

The smallness of the sugar larvae may be thought to result from

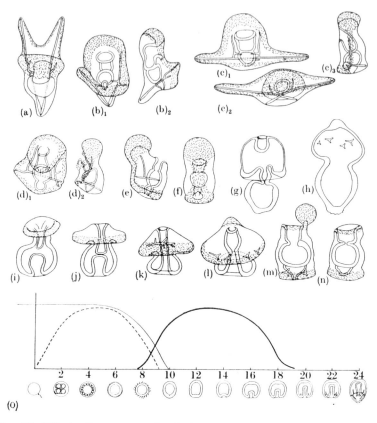

FIG. 56. Effect of sugars on the differentiation of larvae of *Psamm-echinus miliaris*. (a), (b), (d)–(f) Equal parts of sea-water and 0·7 M sucrose, (c) galactose. Combined effect of glucose and 3 per cent (g), (h), or 1·5 per cent (i)–(n) LiCl. While the sensitivity to lithium ions reaches from fertilization to blastula stage (broken line), and to 8-chloroxanthine begins before fertilization (continuous thin line), the sugar action is restricted to a much later period (heavy line). (From Hörstadius 1959.)

shrinking, but it is due rather to lack of the dorsal part and the large amount of material that is tied up in the much enlarged ciliated band. That the sugar effect is not ascribable to shrinking but is of a distinctive nature is obvious from the following. Animal halves showed more or less extended tufts. The sugar effect on whole eggs was attained both with hyper- and hypotonic sugar solutions. The question arises whether the sugar effect is due to changes in electrolytes because of osmotic processes. In all solutions there is a deficit of electrolytes which predisposes to an extrusion from the larva. On the other hand, Bäckström *et al.* (1960)

have shown that glucose labelled with C^{14} can penetrate into sea-urchin larvae. A crucial experiment proving that sugar is indeed capable of exerting a specific effect was made by combining it with lithium. Our figures (g) and (h) represent typical lithium exogastrulae as regards the endoderm. However, the thick acron plate in (h) and the stomodaeum in (g) are differentiations alien to the lithium control larvae. Still more aberrant are the larvae with transverse ciliated band and stomodaeum (i), (j), in (j) of unusual length, invaginating from the animal pole. In (l) and (m) the mouth lies a little to the side of the acron thickening. The larvae (m) and (n) resemble radialized larvae (Fig. 55(b)$_6$, (b)$_7$, (d), (e)), but the size of the digestive tract in relation to the ectoderm is different.

Eggs can be radialized by treatment with 8-chloroxanthine before fertilization (Fig. 56(o)). Experiments were made to test whether such conversion is irrevocable (Hörstadius 1961). Normal meridional halves fused with radialized meridional halves gave normal plutei; normal vegetal halves were able to force back bilateral symmetry upon radialized animal halves. The reciprocal combination, radialized vegetal half fused with normal animal half, did not give clear-cut results. Further experiments are necessary.

8 Experiments at later stages. Bilateral asymmetry

Echinoidea

DRIESCH believed that all blastomeres had equal potencies, the egg being an harmonious equipotential system. In a paper written in 1895, he set himself the task of discovering at what stage the parts cease to be equivalent as regards prospective potencies. He cut up blastulae of *Sphaerechinus granularis* and *Asterias glacialis* into fragments. The operations, however, were made at random on a great mass of blastulae in a drop of sea-water, and the origin of the fragments—that is, their presumptive fate in the whole larva—was not known, nor were any two fragments of the same egg reared together. Although not all of the hundred or so fragments became gastrulae or later stages, Driesch drew the conclusion that all parts of the blastulae were equipotential and totipotent. He then proceeded to perform the same experiments with gastrulae. Isolated ectoderm could not gastrulate, nor could isolated endoderm renew ectoderm. However, Driesch found that within the limits of each germ layer the parts remained equipotential, at least for a time. A part of the archenteron, for example, can form coelom, mesenchyme, and a tripartite gut, but later this becomes impossible.

The problem concerning the stage of determination in gastrulae was dealt with by Jenkinson (1911a) who used a perfect technique, dividing them individually at the desired level, and rearing the two halves together. He arrived at the same result as later was found valid even for cleavage stages—namely, that two complete larvae cannot be obtained after transverse section (see page 71), nor can the archenteron form an equipotential system since not all of its parts are capable of forming a tripartite digestive tract: only parts larger than half of the archenteron can do so. Moreover, there are polar differences as to the faculty of forming coelom and intestine. These early findings of Jenkinson conform rather with the idea of gradients.

The coelomic sac budded off at the tip of the archenteron divides into a left and a right vesicle, growing down along the sides of the alimentary canal (Fig. 57(a)$_1$, (a)$_2$). In each we can distinguish three parts constituting left and right anterior, middle, and posterior coelom. The left posterior coelom (*lpc*) and the right posterior coelom (*rpc*) (a)$_2$ will enclose the stomach and form the hypogastric and epigastric coelom. The left

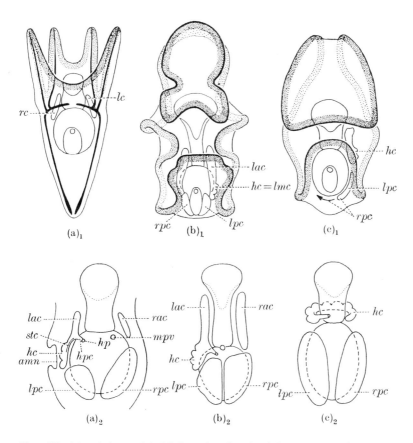

FIG. 57. (a)$_1$ pluteus, (b)$_1$ bipinnaria of a starfish, (c)$_1$ auricularia of a holothurian (all seen from the ventral side). (a)$_2$–(c)$_2$ Interior organs of later stages, as seen from the dorsal side. *amn*, amnion; *hc*, hydrocoele; *hp*, hydropore; *lac*, left anterior coelom; *lc*, left coelom; *lmc*, left middle coelom; *lpc*, left posterior coelom; *mpv*, madreporic vesicle; *rac*, right anterior coelom; *rc*, right coelom; *rpc*, right posterior coelom; *stc*, stone canal.

middle coelom (*lmc*) is the hydrocoele (*hc*) and will soon form five pockets, the rudiments of the radial canals of the water vascular system, whereas the right middle coelom becomes reduced. From the left anterior coelom (*lac*) a tube projects towards the dorsal ectoderm and opens through the primary hydropore (*hp*). The stone canal (*stc*) arises as a groove in the wall of the anterior coelom from the hydrocoele to the hydroporic canal, thus establishing the connexion of the water vascular system with the exterior. Before metamorphosis the ectoderm makes a large invagination outside the hydrocoele (*amn*). This pocket closes, forming the amnion (vestibule), the bottom of which gives rise to the ectodermal tissues of the oral side of the sea-urchin. The disk of hydrocoele and amniotic ectoderm with the presumptive adult mouth in the centre has been called the echinus rudiment. During metamorphosis the larval arms, mouth, oesophagus, and intestine are reduced and resorbed.

Runnström (1915–18, 1925*b*) carried out a series of analytical studies on differentiated sea-urchin larvae. Parts of plutei were cut off with a knife. A new method used to study potencies in old larvae was to starve them and subsequently feed them again (1917) and to reduce their vitality by adding $ZnSO_4$ to the sea-water (1917), or to rear larvae in K- and Mg-free sea-water with increased Ca-content (1925*b*).

Many exceptions to the dominating asymmetry with the hydrocoele on the left side have been reported in echinoderm larvae. Müller depicted an ophiurid larva with two hydrocoeles in 1848, and in 1849 a holothurian auricularia with inverse asymmetry. For literature in this field see Runnström 1918*a*, p. 410; Hörstadius 1928, p. 164). As to sea-urchins, amnion invagination was found in many cases on the right side in connexion with situs inversus of the hydrocoele, and on both sides in plutei with two hydrocoeles. The problem of possible mutual relations for appearance and differentiation of these two organs was studied by Runnström (1917). In larvae fed after a period of starvation, the two components of the echinus rudiment could vary with regard to time, place, or stage of development. From such cases he deduced that the invagination is a self-differentiation as it can appear independently of a hydrocoele. However, the further differentiation of the bottom of the amnion can occur only in contact with the hydrocoele. In contrast, growth of the hydrocoele is released by contact with the bottom of the amnion.

More light was shed upon this early example of dependent differentiation by the study of abnormal larvae isolated from large cultures:

plutei with two amniotic invaginations, with two hydrocoeles, with both rudiments on the right side, with hydrocoele and amnion on opposite sides, or without amnion (1918*a*). The character of self-differentiation of the invagination was confirmed, but a hydrocoele could influence the direction of the ingrowth. On the other hand, the releasing effect of the amniotic bottom on the hydrocoele was not entirely specific as in two cases the hydrocoele was observed to differentiate below other parts of ectoderm.

In the sea-urchin *Genocidaris maculata* the amnion first appears as a compact group of ectoderm cells at considerable distance from the coelomic rudiments (von Ubisch 1959). Its transformation into a vesicle

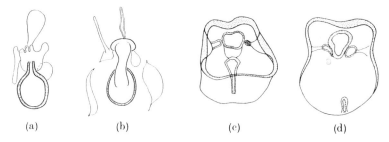

(a)   (b)   (c)   (d)

FIG. 58. (a), (b) Coelomic vesicles protruding from starved and re-fed sea-urchin larvae. (c), (d) Coelom vesicles invaginated from the ectoderm. (From Runnström 1917, 1925*b*.)

is rather slow and as it moves towards the hydrocoele both differentiate in the proper way. In this species also with the aberrant start of amnion formation the character of self-differentiation at the first step was illustrated by observation of larvae with amnion on both left and right sides, in spite of the absence of a right hydrocoele.

In starved and re-fed larvae the formation of coelomic organs takes place in an atypical way (Runnström 1917). A new hydrocoele was able to regenerate from an anterior coelom. In several cases a number of thin-walled vesicles protruded from the oesophagus (Fig. 58(a)). The interpretation of the pouches must be rather arbitrary. In the case illustrated in Fig. 58(b) the conditions are, however, fairly clear. In the larva the anterior coelom and hydrocoele had been completely resorbed, but the posterior coeloms remained. From the oesophagus emanated an elongated pulsating sac, evidently a madreporic vesicle (*mpv* in Fig. 57(a)$_2$), and a left and a right sac, interpreted as hydrocoeles. As to the left sac, there seems to be no doubt since it has a long hydroporic canal with an opening in the ectoderm. The anterior part of the endodermal component of the oesophagus in a pluteus corresponds to the tip of the archenteron from which the coelom normally is budded off. These sacs represent a second formation from the same region. However, regeneration from quite atypical sources is also reported. Migratory cells could gather and fuse into a new madreporic vesicle (1917) or into a posterior coelom (1918*a*). In larvae with diminutive archenteron, coelomic vesicles were obtained (Fig. 58(c, d)) after invagination from the ectoderm on both sides of the mouth (1925*b*). The observations thus disclosed the faculty of forming new coelomic vesicles from coelom, oesophagus, ectoderm, and mesenchyme.

Czihak (1965*a*) killed parts of the left coelom as well as the amnion rudiment by localized ultra-violet radiation. Complete destruction of the left coelom at its formation from the tip of the archenteron led to compensation from the right coelom. This substitute could form hydrocoele and echinus rudiment. A destroyed left posterior coelom could regenerate from hydrocoele or stone canal. On the other hand, while a hydrocoele could not grow out from the *lpc*, it could do so from the stone canal. In contrast, a hydrocoele could give rise to a new stone canal. Destruction on the left side never resulted in hydrocoele formation on the right side. These local disengagements of the left coelom or parts thereof have led to replacements only within the coelom system itself and not from other germ layers as in the experiments by Runnström or in those reported on starfish and holothurians in the next Sections. Amnion also was destroyed by radiation. The ectoderm could form a new invagination also in the absence of a hydrocoele, a confirmation of the findings just mentioned that the amnion can appear independently of the hydrocoele.

Arms or the apex with the body-rods were removed by sections at different angles (Runnström 1915). As a consequence of the operation, skeleton spicules sometimes initially decreased in number but a regeneration followed. Skeleton-forming mesenchyme cells in great numbers left their rods and moved to the point of regeneration, which sometimes manifested growth in an atypical direction and led to the formation of a protuberance on the body-wall giving rise to incomplete twin structures; these could, however, be incorporated by regulation. If a new mouth was formed, its position was determined by the median plane of the larva. The capacity of regulation was found to be greater in later than in early stages of larval development. The statement that an isolated piece of ectoderm including a small part of an epaulette could form endoderm and change polarity is surprising (Fig. 59).

Larvae considerably inhibited in differentiation by starvation were found to produce pedicellariae prematurely in relation to other organs (Runnström 1917). It was impossible to remove the amnion by operation: plutei deprived of amnion could, however, be obtained by removal of left arms which resulted in reduction of not only amnion but also hydrocoele (1918*b*). Some larvae were isolated in which for some reason an amnion had not developed or had been resorbed. In such larvae Runnström (1918*b*) discovered organs which are not expected to occur in sea-urchin larvae. In plutei, the intestine acts as the excretory organ. In

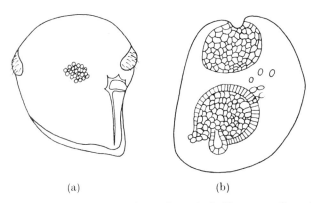

(a)   (b)

FIG. 59. (a) An isolated piece of ectoderm including a small part of an epaulette and a spicule from an old pluteus has regenerated endoderm (b). (From Runnström 1915.)

some larvae without echinus rudiment, small bulges of coelomic vesicles contained granules of excretory character kept in motion by cilia. In one larva a real excretory organ was found (Fig. 60(a)). It consisted of a long tube which opened into the intestine; in the lumen of the terminal part the cilia held the granules in rotation. Excretory granules were also observed in cells of the wall, which was surrounded by mesenchyme cells. In one larva the ectoderm near the anus was evaginated (Fig. 60(b)$_1$). The cells of the epithelium (b)$_2$ produced a sticky substance by which the larva attached itself to the bottom. This fixing organ was partly destroyed when the larva was removed from the glass, but it regenerated.

Runnström (1917) explains the premature appearance of pedicellariae as caused by the disappearance of an inhibiting action in starving larvae normally exercised by other developing organs. Particularly noteworthy is the development of the larval excretory organ, as well as of the fixing organ, as this latter type is found only in starfish and crinoids among the echinoderms. In these cases it was also assumed that phylogenetically old existing potencies are inhibited in the course of normal development (1918*b*).

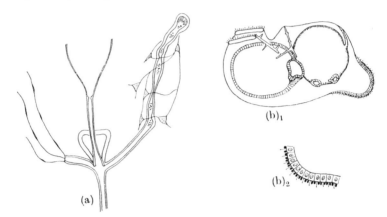

FIG. 60. (a) Development of an excretory organ in an old pluteus without amnion. One larva evaginated a fixing organ, (b)$_1$, its epithelium producing a sticky substance, (b)$_2$. (From Runnström 1918*b*.)

Asteroidea

Among the starfish there are two different types of larval development. Larvae emanating from small eggs, 100–200 μm, are free-swimming up to metamorphosis and depending on uptake of food, while larvae from large eggs pass through an abridged development and rely entirely on their yolk enclosures. The starfish larvae differ from those of sea-urchins in having neither primary mesenchyme nor skeleton.

Schaxel (1914) isolated blastomeres of *Asterias glacialis* using Ca-free sea-water and stated that meridional fragments of 2- and 4-cell stages as well as vegetal cells of 8-cell stages are able to form dwarf larvae, while animal cells do not gastrulate.

The swimming transparent starfish larvae are called bipinnariae (see Fig. 57(b). The anterior–ventral part of the ciliated band encircles a preoral field. The larvae of the genus *Astropecten* remain bipinnariae up to metamorphosis when the larval body is resorbed. The bipinnariae of *Asterias* change to a brachiolaria stage shortly before metamorphosis by forming an attachment organ at the front end. The larvae of *Luidia* swim by muscular contractions of the very large preoral part which at metamorphosis sloughs off. The differentiation of the inner organs is, in principle, the same as in sea-urchins (Fig. 57(b)$_2$).

The body of the larva with abridged development is round or barrel-shaped; the anterior preoral part forms a large fixing organ, stretched in dorsal and ventral directions (Fig. 61(e)). Experiments on such larvae are presented first. After transverse section of young *Asterina gibbosa* gastrulae (Hörstadius 1925*a*, 1928) (see Fig. 61(a), I) animal halves formed a preoral lobe with sucker while the vegetal half, containing the packet of internal organs, formed a reduced sucker and in other respects developed as a complete larva. Removed animal ectoderm (a, II) could be histologically differentiated as a sucker. When the preoral lobe was

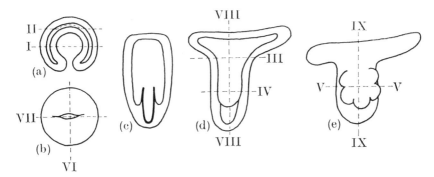

FIG. 61. *Asterina gibbosa.* (a) Longitudinal optical section of gastrula. (b) Gastrula viewed from the vegetal pole. (c) Horizontal section of 4-day-old larva. Heavy line, primitive gut enclosed by coelom pockets. (d) 4-day-old larva from the left with preoral lobe. (e) 6-day-old larva with the five ambulacral rudiments. I–IX, plane of sections. (From Hörstadius 1928.)

removed in older larvae (4 days, (d, III)) no sucker regenerated. The larvae then began to swim, which they otherwise never do, following a spiral course like other echinoderm larvae. They passed through metamorphosis without a sessile stage. Four- and 6-day old larvae were divided by a cut across the hydrocoele ((d, IV), (e, V)); both fragments were able to develop into small starfish in which the missing rays could postgenerate. This last result may seem to be contrary to the observations made in the study of sea-urchins where no egg or early larva could give rise to two larvae after having been divided by a transverse section (see p. 71). The experiments with bipinnariae and auriculariae point in the same direction (see later). It must be stressed, however, that in the work reported in this chapter we were unable to use early cleavage stages. As to the development of the fragments obtained by sectioning, along lines IV and V no complete larval bodies were obtained. Only the

animal part has a fixing organ. In these larvae with abridged development it is in fact the starfish rudiment which is divided and which has
reached a stage allowing continued differentiation and even regeneration.
Note the immense regenerative capacity of starfish.

As regards experiments with left and right halves, the first paper in
the field (Runnström 1920) is of special interest because it introduces
the methods of transplantation and constriction on echinoderm material.
The experiments with eggs of *Henricia sanguinolenta* and *Solaster*
(species not known) were somewhat hampered by lack of material. They
were continued by isolation experiments on larvae of *Asterina gibbosa*
(Hörstadius 1925a, 1928). Contrary to earlier statements the cleavage
stages of *Henricia* and *Solaster* allowed an orientation with regard to egg
axis and plane of symmetry. In *Asterina* the shape of the blastopore
offered a similar possibility.

Cleavage stages of *Henricia* with 60–100 blastomeres were divided
into left and right halves (Runnström 1920), of which one was rotated
through 180° and transplanted back on the other half. Invagination
started at both vegetal poles and gave rise to two more or less complete
internal twins, but, as a rule, only one sucker developed. Both dorsal
and ventral halves contain rudiments of both left and right coelomic
vesicles. Frontal constriction in early cleavage stages (*Henricia*) or in
gastrulae (*Solaster*) resulted accordingly in reduplication of hydrocoele
and sucker (Runnström 1920). After complete separation (at gastrula
stage, *Asterina*, see Fig. 61(b, VII)) both halves developed into complete
larvae, although the skeleton on the aboral side was defective at least in
one partner. In all cases the hydrocoele belonged to the original left side.

Complete separation of early left and right halves as well as a few cases
of median constriction revealed that left halves have a higher viability
(*Asterina*, (b, VI)). They always developed a typical hydrocoele on their
left side. However, the skeleton on the new right, future aboral, side
was more or less delayed and defective. Rather few of the right partners
reached full differentiation, but in the *Asterina* material it could be
stated that they may form a hydrocoele on their presumptive left or right
side, or on both sides, as illustrated in Fig. 62(a), (c), (b). Starfish obtained
after metamorphosis of right halves had only three or four ambulacral
rays and a correspondingly incomplete oral and aboral skeleton (c).
Larvae with two hydrocoeles (b) or without hydrocoele had cylindrical
body and skeletal plates of aboral type irregularly distributed. The
faculty of forming skeletal plates seems to be inherent in the body-wall,
but their type and pattern depend on the hydrocoele. Isolated left and

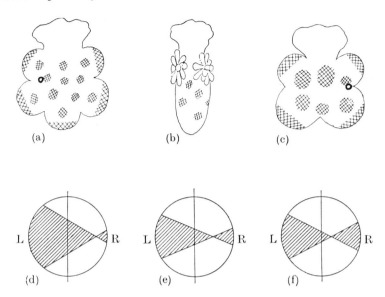

FIG. 62. *Asterina gibbosa.* (a) A left half, (c) a right half, both seen from the aboral side. The position of the madrepore indicates that the hydrocoele of the left half had developed at its left side, that of the right half on its right side. (b) A right half with double hydrocoele. (d)–(f) Tentative explanation of formation of hydrocoele on the left side, on both sides, or on the right side in right halves. (From Hörstadius 1928.)

right halves of 4-day-old larvae (stage shown in Fig. 61(d)) have lost the capacity of replacing missing coelomic organs. A left half will metamorphose without epigastric coelom, but in compensation a branch of the hypogastric coelom takes its place. The right halves develop no hydrocoele and therefore the body remains cylindrical.

It has been shown that meridional halves of different origin, by regulation in early development, can compensate for the missing parts. By postgeneration the reduced number of ambulacral rays can be completed. Will reorganization take place if two left or two right halves are fused? This question was answered by Runnström (1920). Two left and two right halves of late gastrulae of *Henricia* were brought together. In both combinations each side differentiated as it should have done—that is, the larvae had two ambulacral (Fig. 63(a)) and two aboral sides. However, although the transplantation was carried out at such a late stage a certain regulation was observed. The sucker normally has a longer dorsal and a shorter ventral branch. In the larva (Fig. 63(a)), however, they both have the same orientation as a consequence of an adaptation of one of the rudiments to the new unit. In some cases one side took the lead in the subsequent development, and increased its ambulacral system, whereas it became inhibited on the other side, which instead began to develop the character of an aboral side with spines. Of particular interest is the larva in Fig. 63(b), consisting of two fused right halves. These formed two aboral sides with skeletal plates, but in the region of fusion an ambulacral system with three rays was postgenerated. This grew to become a real oral side under an aboral side of double origin (b)$_2$.

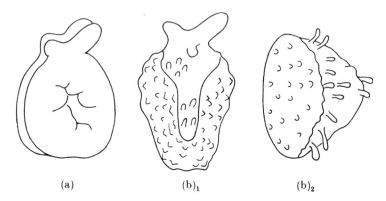

(a)   (b)$_1$ (b)$_2$

Fig. 63. *Henricia sanguinolenta.* (a), Fusion of two left (ambulacral) halves of late gastrula stages. (b)$_1$ After fusion of two right halves some ambulacral feet developed in the region of fusion. (b)$_2$ In the course of development the ambulacral field increased, leading to a little starfish with three ambulacral rows and peculiar double aboral side. (From Runnström 1920.)

On the basis of some observations of echinoderm larvae with two hydrocoeles, Runnström (1918a, p. 427) assumed that asymmetry is present even in the uncleaved egg and is caused by the asymmetric distribution of promoting and inhibiting substances and metabolic processes. A tentative explanation of quantitative relations in association with a double gradient theory is given in Fig. 62(d)–(f).

Experimental studies on larvae of starfish with a long free-swimming life have been carried out on gastrulae and bipinnariae of *Astropecten aranciacus* (Hörstadius 1925b, 1928, normal development 1939b). The fertilization membrane was tough and could not be removed by shaking. The cleavage stages and the markedly folded blastulae did not allow any orientation. Gastrulae and young bipinnariae were divided by transverse cuts, according to the planes I–VII in Fig. 64. The animal half of the ectoderm (I, IV) produced blastulae with, in some cases, a piece of ciliated band and small stomodaeum. When the section was laid across the dilated end of the archenteron (II) from which the coelomic sacs later detach, the animal fragments differentiated as the corresponding part of a bipinnaria, with preoral band, mouth and two small coeloms. The vegetal partners after isolation along I or II showed mosaic differentiation but had the power of postgenerating the missing organs—preoral band and mouth. The sections laid further vegetally (III) evidently hit different planes. In some cases the results were similar to those described for II; in others the animal fragment grew to a bipinnaria without intestine which, however, could be postgenerated, whereas the vegetal part with intestine only was not capable of reorganization. The middle

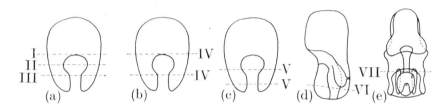

Fɪɢ. 64. *Astropecten aranciacus.* I–VII, plane of isolations in gastrulae (a)–(c), transitional stage (d) to bipinnaria (e). (From Hörstadius 1928.)

region IV–IV formed either a large stomodaeum and a piece of a preoral band, or a small bipinnaria, initially lacking preoral lobe and intestine and with only a small mouth. In accordance with expectations, the fragments V–V developed into bipinnariae without anal opening or preoral field and with only a small mouth, and possessing the faculty of supplementary growth to harmonious shape. The animal parts of 3-day-old (VI) and the vegetal parts of 9-day-old (VII) larvae could also compensate for the losses.

The experiments show that it is not possible to obtain two complete larvae after transverse section. The fragments differentiate in the main according to their prospective significance. Afterwards, a regeneration or postgeneration may set in, but it is only one of the fragments from each larva that can attain the shape of a complete bipinnaria. Only those fragments containing an area of the archenteron just below the coelomic distension possess the requisite potentialities. Such a fragment may have a volume less than half that of the larva. Only in this area, apparently, is there an harmonious balance between animal and vegetal qualities.

Early gastrulae were divided by sections into meridional halves before coelomic bulges of the archenteron tip allowed determination of the ventro–dorsal axis. The ensuing development of the ciliated band showed which halves represented the left and right parts of the larva. They therefore could be expected to form either left or right coelomic sacs. However, a regulation took place. Coelomic vesicles were budded off on both sides, but on the cut side they were delayed and smaller.

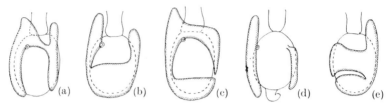

FIG. 65. *Astropecten aranciacus.* (a)–(c), (e) Regeneration of coelom from coelom, (d) from the stomach, in left halves (a)–(d) and in a right half (e). (From Hörstadius 1928.)

Left and right halves of gastrulae were isolated when the ventro–dorsal axis became discernible. Each pair was reared in a separate bowl. The halves then lost the faculty of immediately replacing coelom on the cut side. In all healthy larvae, however, an endeavour towards regeneration of coelom in the coelom-free side was observed. Various courses were taken:

(1) by outgrowths from the left coelom either (i) on the animal side of the hydropore (Fig. 65(a)), or (ii) in the more vegetal part (b), or (iii) by both ways simultaneously (c); in right halves by outgrowths from the right coelom towards the left side (e);

(2) by a bud from the stomach (d); the point belongs to the middle region of the archenteron—compare the origin of coelomic vesicles in sea-urchins from a region corresponding to the tip of the archenteron, the normal coelom-forming part (Fig. 58);

(3) by formation of vesicles by mesenchyme cells (Fig. 66(b));

(4) by an invagination from a supplementary pore in the ectoderm in the neighbourhood of the hydropore.

Several methods could be used at the same time. The following combinations were observed: 1(i) + 1(ii), 1 + 2, 1(ii) + 3. A case of the last type is illustrated in Fig. 66. A madreporic vesicle (*Mp*) and a small coelomic sac (*Cöl*) were formed in a right half by mesenchyme cells (b). The right posterior coelom grew over to the left side, sent a protrusion towards, and fused with, the new coelom (a)–(d). In one series the right coelom of a young bipinnaria was drawn out through a slit in the ectoderm. In 10 cases the regeneration methods (1), (2), and (3) were observed.

The regeneration of coelomic vesicles from different sources is perhaps less astonishing in view of the observations that the madreporic vesicle in *Astropecten* in the course of normal development can arise from mesenchyme cells, from the right middle coelom, or from the ectoderm (see Figs. 24, 25 in Hörstadius 1939*b*).

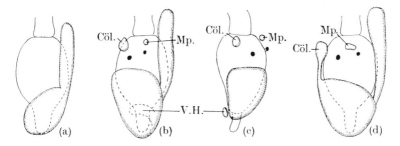

FIG. 66. *Astropecten aranciacus.* A coelomic vesicle formed by mesenchyme cells (*Cöl.*) fused with an outgrowth on the left side from the right posterior coelom (d). (a), (b), (d) From the dorsal side, (c) from the left side. See text for further explanation. (From Hörstadius 1928.)

The material available also provides an answer to the question of asymmetry of hydrocoele-pores in pairs of left and right halves. Of 20 left halves, 18 showed normal asymmetry, while two had pores on both sides. In the right halves all possibilities were represented: left, right, both sides, or none at all—conditions similar to those observed in *Asterina*.

Holothurioidea

The planktonic transparent auricularia (*Holothuria, Synapta*) bears an external resemblance to a bipinnaria, but the preoral field is not completely enclosed as the left and right parts of the ciliated band remain separate also at the animal pole (see Fig. 57(c)$_1$). The difference is more conspicuous in the coelomic system: from the archenteron tip only one vesicle is budded off (Fig. 67(b), (c)); it moves and grows down along the left side of the digestive tract and divides into two parts (Fig. 57(c)$_1$, Fig. 67(d), (e)). The anterior vesicle is the rudiment of the hydrocoele, connected with the exterior by a hydropore and bending around the oesophagus to form the ambulacral ring (Fig. 57(c)$_2$). The posterior part continues towards the posterior pole, stretching and bending around the intestine and following the right side of the stomach

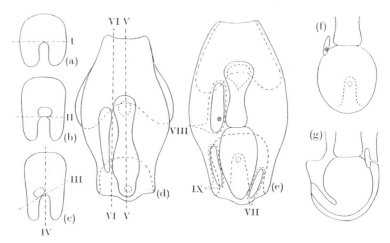

FIG. 67. *Holothuria poli*. I–IX in (a)–(e) indicate the operations on gastrulae and auriculariae. (f), (g) Regeneration of a coelomic vesicle by invagination from a hydropore. (c)–(f) The larvae seen from the dorsal side. (Hörstadius 1928.)

(c)$_1$. The left and right parts are tied off from each other and give rise to the posterior left and right coeloms (Fig. 67(e)).

As it was impossible to rear even whole larvae of *Holothuria poli* to late auriculariae, the life of operated larvae was, of course, also short, but the following observations were achieved (Hörstadius 1925c, 1928). The ectoderm isolated in front of the early archenteron tip (Fig. 67(a), I) formed blastulae with ciliated band. The vegetal part developed into auricularia although with initially too-small animal organs. A section between the coelomic vesicle and the archenteron tip (II and III in (b) and (c)) gave another result. The animal fragment developed a ciliated band and a stomodaeum capable of swallowing movements, and contained the coelom which, however, did not differentiate further. The development of the vegetal half was surprisingly poor. A ciliated band appeared, but the gut could not develop a mouth, which hampered its survival. As in sea-urchins and starfish, left halves had a greater capacity for development than right halves. Left halves of early gastrulae (IV in (c)) reached stages of young auriculariae with typical differentiation of coelomic vesicles. Right halves also reached the shape of auricularia, but without coelom. At the age of 2 days, larvae were divided along the lines V and VI in (d). In some larvae without coelom a hydropore invagination could extend to a small canal. Buds from the stomach were also observed.

In older larvae (3–5 days old) coelomic sacs were drawn out through a slit in the ectoderm. After removal of the right posterior coelom ((e), VII) a substitute could be obtained in the same way as in normal development, by growth from the *lpc* around the intestine. Lack of hydrocoele and *lpc* (VIII, IX) led to attempts at regeneration in several ways: a vesicle invaginated from a hydropore (f), (g), a bud projected from the stomach, a small sac was probably formed by mesenchyme. Fusions of vesicles of these different origins were also seen.

The conditions of regeneration thus show a considerable resemblance to those in starfish. It should be added that in the holothurians, with their pronounced asymmetry, coelom formation in coelom-free right halves always took place on the left side.

Many sea cucumbers have large eggs and pass through an abridged development phase. The cleavage of *Psolus phantapus* and of *Cucumaria frondosa* is of bilateral type, and in *Psolus* the unripe egg as well as blastula and gastrula show a ventro–dorsal structure (Runnström and Runnström 1920). These facts were used for experiments. Shortly after the onset of gastrulation larvae were divided by frontal sections. Both halves gastrulated and formed coelom and hydrocoele. This is according to expectation as both the dorsal and the ventral fragments contain presumptive endoderm and coelom. Elsewhere in the paper the authors correctly speak of halves after frontal sectioning as dorsal and ventral; it is, therefore, surprising that the halves in question are called animal and vegetal, and that the conclusion is drawn that there is no limitation to the capacity of the presumptive ectoderm to form mesoderm and endoderm. This statement, if it really refers to animal and not to dorsal and ventral halves, is incompatible with the findings in other echinoderms, including *Holothuria*. Gastrulae in later stages were also divided in halves, now evidently animal and vegetal. The animal halves contained the front end of the archenteron. Both fragments were capable of developing by postgeneration into more or less typical larvae. A similar faculty of growth characterized animal and vegetal fragments of larvae with vestibule and tentacles. The ambiguous statement on endoderm formation from animal ectoderm requires reinvestigation.

Crinoidea

The majority of the adult Crinoidea are sessile from the stage of fixation of the larva in early life until the end of their life-span. The members of the family *Antedonidae* constitute an exception. The larva develops into a Pentacrinus, attached to the substrate by a long stalk carrying the calyx, which has radial, ramified arms with pinnulae, and cirri at the base, but the adult detaches itself from the stalk to a swimming life. The development of several species of *Antedonidae* has been described by a number of embryologists (Carpenter 1866; Barrois 1888; Bury 1888; Perrier 1889; Seeliger 1892; Mortensen 1920).

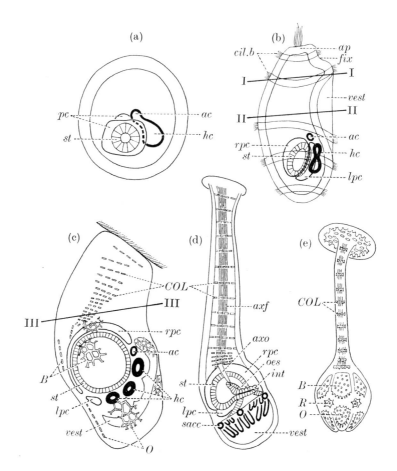

FIG. 68. *Antedon rosacea.* (a) Gastrula with coelomic vesicles. (b) Swimming larva with ciliated bands, fixation pit and rudiment of vestibule. (c) Fixed larva with closed vestibule and developing calcareous ossicles. (d), (e) Later stages. I–III, planes of sections. *ac*, anterior coelom; *ap*, apical plate; *axf*, axial fibres; *axo*, axial organ; *B*, basalia; *cil.b*, ciliated band; *COL*, columnalia; *fix*, fixation pit; *hc*, hydrocoele; *int*, intestine; *lpc*, left posterior coelom; *O*, oralia; *oes*, oesophagus; *pc*, posterior coelom; *R*, radialia; *rpc*, right posterior coelom; *sacc*, sacculus; *st*, stomach; *vest*, vestibule. ((a)–(d) Redrawn from Seeliger 1892; (e) After Thomson 1865.)

The early larva is barrel-shaped. It has an apical plate with a tuft, and a larval nervous system is connected with the plate. The body has five transverse ciliated bands which serve as swimming organs (Fig. 68(b)). After invagination the archenteron in a somewhat complicated way gives rise to a sac-like gut without an opening but from which the oesophagus and intestine subsequently develop. Two coelomic vesicles cover the sides of the gut (a). They correspond to the left and right posterior coeloms of other echinoderms (*pc* in (a)). A third vesicle consists of a smaller anterior part, the parietal canal (*ac*) which will open through the ectodermal primary madreporic pore, and a larger posterior part, also lying close to the gut, the hydrocoele (*hc*). The stone canal is formed in the wall of the channel between the parietal canal and the hydrocoele. The parietal canal and the hydrocoele are considered to be equivalent to left anterior and middle coelomic vesicles of other echinoderms.

There is a small glandular pit in the ectoderm in a gap in the first ciliated band. This is the fixation pit by which the larva attaches itself to the substratum ((b) *fix*). At the same time and on the same side a large sac is invaginated between the second and third rings: the vestibule (*vest*). After fixation the anterior part of the larva is transformed into a long stalk, stiffened by calcareous ossicles (foot-plate, columnal plates, *COL*). The free end of the elongated larva thus corresponds to the blastoporic pole. The invagination opening of the vestibule is closed. The inner wall of the ectodermal sac formed in this way is pressed against the packet of the gut and coelomic vesicles, and contributes to the formation of tentacles and mouth. Initially the vestibule and hydrocoele evidently are oriented laterally. Then the whole complex begins to rotate until the oral side faces the free end. The vestibule opens and the arms grow out. The rotating movement has been called elevation.

In the free-swimming larvae two rows, each consisting of five skeletal plates, orals and basals, form slightly oblique rings around the body (c), (e). In the sessile Pentacrinus they now represent transverse rings, the orals between the outgrowing arms, the basals close to the stalk (e). The skeleton is thus from the outset more adjusted to the adult radial symmetry than are the rotating vestibule-inner organs. Between orals and basals are found the five sacculi, which are clumps of mesenchyme cells (d).

Abnormal larvae have been described by several authors (Barrois, Seeliger, Mortensen). In these cases the larvae had failed to attach themselves, or their fixation-time had for some reason been too short. In such larvae the closure and the rotation of the vestibule had been checked, but in spite of that a differentiation could occur. An experimental analysis of determination was made by Runnström (1925a). He started from the fact that the attachment involves a turning-point in development. Ciliated band, glandular cells, and the larval nervous system become resorbed. On the other hand, all the other processes connected with elevation occur. Runnström, therefore, studied the effect of checking fixation by removing the front end of the larva.

Swimming larvae were divided with a scalpel into anterior and posterior parts by cuts made approximately along the lines I–I and II–II

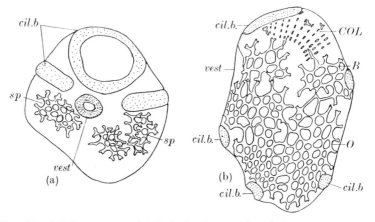

FIG. 69. *Antedon rosacea.* (a) Anterior fragment and (b) posterior fragment of a swimming larva. *B*, basalia; *cil.b*, ciliated band; *COL*, columnalia; *O*, oralia; *sp*, skeletal plate; *vest*, vestibule. (From Runnström 1925a.)

in Fig. 68(b). The anterior parts generally attached themselves to the substrate. A stalk-like elongation did not occur, as might have been expected (Fig. 69(a)). The fixation pit became reduced, but the apical plate and the larval nervous system remained unaffected. The ciliated bands also remained, or their disappearance was considerably delayed. A vestibular sac was invaginated. The development of the skeletal plates was rather unexpected. Only few, if any, stalk ossicles (columnalia) were observed. On the other hand, a pentamerous ring of plates resembling oralia and basalia, thus calyx plates, developed in the isolated stalk fragment (a). In the posterior parts neither fixation pit nor larval nervous system appeared. The free-swimming larvae kept their oval form (b). Here also the reduction of ciliated band was delayed. In most cases the opening of the vestibule did not close. Even if it did so, no rotation of vestibule and interior organs took place. Sacculae could be formed independently of elevation. The calcareous plates became arranged in a fairly typical way independently of other organs but sometimes fused (b). Both coelomic vesicles and gut could be more or less doubled. If thereby two hydrocoeles appeared, the left, as a rule, was better developed than the right. A certain differentiation of the hydrocoele could take place without connexion with the exterior through a canal and pore. Tentacle buds were observed also when the hydrocoele had no contact with the vestibule.

Fixed larvae were sectioned along the line III–III in Fig. 68(c) shortly after the attachment, as well as two days later. The anterior fragments then developed into elongated stalks with a largely typical skeleton, thus constituting a differentiation quite divergent from that of the anterior parts isolated in the early stages.

The posterior parts were capable of developing into calices with tentacles protruding through an open vestibule and with typical skeleton of oralia and basalia. No regeneration of a stalk ensued. The great number of reduplications of inner organs and also of vestibules was striking. Runnström states that on twinning gut arises from gut and posterior coelom also from corresponding tissue, but he leaves open the question of the origin of hydrocoele and parietal canal.

From the reports mentioned above of earlier authors on abnormal larvae, and from his own experiments, Runnström formed the opinion that fixation is a prerequisite of rotation of vestibule and inner organs. However, his later observations based on extensive material led him to the conclusion that fixation is not necessary for a normal course of metamorphosis (1930). As to causal explanation of the processes, he states that the rotation does not depend on the ectoderm, but is due rather to the mesenchyme in connexion with changes in internal pressure. The fixation of the larva and the almost immediately following reduction of ciliated bands, larval nervous system, and gland cells in the ectoderm, as well as the closing of the vestibule and the inflation of the gut, led him to assume that hormones form in the anterior region. The fact that isolated anterior parts do not reduce their ciliated bands and larval nervous system speaks rather for hormonal production in the posterior part. This incompatibility is explained by Runnström's assumption that the hormones formed in the anterior part first have to interact with substances in the posterior part. The vestibule invagination is independent of the hydrocoele which forms five lobes independently of the vestibule, but an interaction is necessary for further differentiation.

Progressive determination

For lack of experimental data the distribution of potencies and state
of determination are not known in uncleaved eggs and in early cleavage
stages of starfish, sea cucumbers, and sea lilies. Nevertheless, some of
the isolation experiments illustrate a progressive determination. Vegetal
halves of early gastrulae of *Asterina* could regenerate a sucker, although
small, but this capacity was lost at the age of four days. The animal
halves of swimming *Antedon* larvae attached themselves but did not
elongate as a stalk. They formed few, if any, columnalia. Instead, they
developed plates of calyx type, which represented a differentiation in
the direction of a whole. On the other hand, in corresponding fragments
of older fixed larvae the determination led to a development in accordance with their prospective significance—a long stalk with proper
footplate and columnalia.

Right halves of early gastrulae of *Asterina* could develop a hydrocoele
on their left or right side, or on both sides (see Fig. 62), but right halves
derived from 4-day-old larvae were not capable of forming a new hydrocoele. As regards the species with transparent swimming larvae it was
found that both left and right halves of early gastrulae (*Astropecten*)
sometimes budded off a coelomic sac from the tip of the archenteron on
the cut side, although the process was delayed and the sac was smaller.
In halves isolated at the late gastrula stage the regeneration had to take
other paths.

It was early observed that the material from which primary organs
are derived in embryonic development was arranged in layers. In 1828
von Baer pointed out that homologous structures in various animals
are formed of material from corresponding layers. This germ-layer
conception, valuable for systematizing facts, was soon considered a
'law', although it was based on insufficient morphological data and was
never tested experimentally. A sensation was created at the end of the
past century when a number of observations showed that mesenchyme
in the vertebrate head as well as the pigment cells originate from the
neural crest—thus from the ectoderm (Platt 1893; Borcea 1909; lit. in
Hörstadius 1950). How untenable this old notion is stands out clearly
also from the experiments described earlier. It is remarkable how larvae
perceive the lack of coelom and try to compensate for its loss by different methods. In sea-urchins regeneration or postgeneration is reported
from coelom, mesenchyme, oesophagus, and ectoderm. In *Astropecten*
the observations include coelom, mesenchyme, stomach and ectoderm,

and sometimes two methods at the same time. Similar phenomena have been noted in larvae of *Holothuria*.

In plutei—that is in larvae with the embryonic differentiation accomplished—the power of regeneration or postgeneration was found to have increased. A minor ectodermal fragment was found to produce endoderm (see Fig. 59). Old starving larvae were capable of producing an atypical excretory organ and even of evaginating a fixing organ (see Fig. 60), differentiations entirely unknown in sea-urchin larvae.

Reference has been made to the literature on echinoderm larvae which reported hydrocoele on both sides, proof that the right middle coelom also has a dormant faculty that can be brought into action and thereby do away with the asymmetry. In this chapter it has been shown that the potency is often revived in isolated right halves leading to larvae with only right hydrocoele or with hydrocoele on both sides (see Fig. 62). Larvae with two hydrocoeles or with *situs inversus* have also been obtained by rearing in sea-water with alterations in salinity. MacBride (1918) and Ohshima (1922) transferred sea-urchin larvae aged between 3 and 4 days into hypertonic sea-water and found right hydrocoele in a few of the plutei. However, these are not, as in the isolation experiments, cases of changed embryonic differentiation, but a secondary phenomenon: the inversion probably depends on closure of the left hydropore, which led to a postgeneration on the right side. Runnström (1925c) instead used hypotonic sea-water, and from the beginning of development. In a series of 390 3-day-old larvae he found only 16 per cent with normal asymmetry. Strange to say, the majority formed only one coelom rudiment, and of these only 10 per cent had it on the left as against 12 per cent on the right side. In more than half the series the sole sac was either ventral or dorsal, which represented a considerable variation from the normal. In some of these larvae a tendency towards restoration of normal symmetry was observed in the growth and division of the coelomic vesicle.

9 *Sea-urchins and genetics*

TODAY the historical perspective of many fundamental facts in genetics has been lost. That the individuality of chromosomes persists during interphase, that egg and sperm carry about the same set of chromosomes, that chromosomes are qualitatively different as carriers of genetic material are all considered obvious. Few remember, and many fail to ponder on the ingenious basic investigations which brought us this knowledge. The great name in this context is Theodor Boveri.

Several authors in the 1880s expressed the opinion that the nuclei, and particularly the chromosomes, were carriers of heredity. Several observations on sea-urchins supported the concept of the decisive role of the nucleus—as, for example, when the sperm nucleus from another species failed to fuse with the egg nucleus until in one of the two first blastomeres the haploid half of the larva showed maternal characters while the other half developed as a hybrid: apart from the cytoplasm of the sperm, this result was interpreted as an indication of activity of the sperm nucleus. A proof that in the egg also the nucleus and not the cytoplasm contained hereditary substance was sought in eggs with an abnormal size relationship of nucleus to cytoplasm. Unfertilized eggs after treatment with CO_2 or NH_3 could form spindles but only monasters, leading to eggs with nucleus of double or quadruple size. After fertilization with sperm from another species the larvae became markedly matrocline; although the male chromosomes had not been eliminated, they were more matrocline than ordinary hybrids. (Herbst 1906*b*, 1909, 1912, 1913, 1914, 1926; Hinderer 1914; Landauer 1922.) The size relations in the above-mentioned experiments indicate that the direction of inheritance depends on the amount of sexual nuclei present.

To fulfil the task as carrier of heredity, continuity is necessary, but the individuality of the chromosomes seemed to vanish in interphase. However, Boveri (1887) demonstrated in *Ascaris* that they also remain in the diffuse state.

Understanding of fertilization was increased by Boveri's (1890) statements that in sea-urchins the centriole is brought by the sperm, and that egg nucleus and sperm nucleus carry the same number of chromosomes. By establishing the individuality of the chromosomes and their regular occurrence in egg and sperm, the probability of their function as heredity material was much strengthened, though not proved. Another open question was whether each chromosome contained the whole mass of genetic factors, or was qualitatively different. The desired proof as well as the answer to this problem was given by the study of sea-urchin eggs fertilized by two sperms—dispermy (Boveri 1902, 1908).

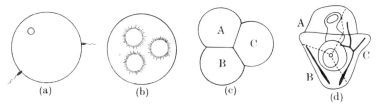

Fig. 70. (a) Egg fertilized by two sperms. (b) Triaster stage, resulting in (c) three blastomeres. (d) Pluteus with three regions showing different degrees of differentiation. (After Boveri 1908.)

When there is a great excess of sperm, the block against polyspermy sometimes fails to function. The entry into the egg of two sperms each bringing a centriole results in the appearance of three (Fig. 70(b)) or four radiating centres with between them three or four spindles—the triaster and tetraster stages. The egg then has three sets of haploid chromosomes. Before it simultaneously divides into three or four blastomeres, the chromosomes are distributed into three or four groups. It is evident that the three sets cannot give rise to four daughter-nuclei with a complete number of chromosomes. Even in triasters it is not very likely that the three cells would receive exactly the right chromosomes and perform a normal differentiation. The haploid number in the sea-urchins varies somewhat with the species: in *Paracentrotus* it is 18. It was mathematically calculated that with triasters only 11 per cent of the cells would receive all types of chromosomes, and in tetrasters such a distribution would hardly ever occur. Boveri found only 79 normal plutei among 719 isolated three-cell stages (about 11 per cent) and only one pluteus from 1500 simultaneous four-cell embryos (1902, 1908).

Within the series from plutei to quite abnormal development, Boveri found larvae with a mosaic of regions showing varying degrees of differentiation. In a larva like the one in Fig. 70(d) the regions corresponding to the blastomeres A–C could be identified. By this ingenious method Boveri proved not only that the chromosomes are carriers of heredity, but also that they are qualitatively different, as atypical distribution brings abnormalities. Baltzer (1910) found that crosses of *Paracentrotus lividus* ♀ × *Sphaerechinus granularis* ♂ give intermediate hybrids while retaining all their chromosomes. However, in the reciprocal combination the larvae either show mainly maternal characters or turn abnormal, evidently because a number of the *Sphaerechinus* chromosomes become eliminated. The qualitative differences were proved by the observation that some recognizable chromosomes in such cases either remained or were eliminated.

The discovery by Boveri together with contemporary results of breeding experiments, particularly by Sutton in the USA, brought chromosome research into harmony with the results of Mendel and paved the way for Morgan's *Drosophila* school with the detection of linear arrangement of the genes, and, in recent times, of their chemical character. In this connexion it is again tempting to mention Boveri's foresight by a quotation: 'The morphologist also could think of nothing better than a morphological analysis leading to a point at which the final elements are chemical individuals' (translation from the German, 1904b, p. 123).

Boveri (1902, 1914b) also advanced the idea that abnormal mitoses might be the cause of malignant tumours. We know that some types of tumours can be induced by virus. Recent investigations on cell hybridization, however, have also given support to Boveri's hypothesis. After treatment with a virus inactivated by ultraviolet radiation the cytoplasm of adjacent cells from different organs, and even from different species, can be brought to complete coalescence. The virus most commonly used is the Sendai virus, a member of the parainfluenza group of myxoviruses. Multinucleated cells may be formed. In binucleated cells the two nuclei fuse at mitosis. After cell division, two daughter cells are obtained, each containing in its nucleus the chromosomes of both parent cells. These mononucleate cells are capable of multiplication for many generations even when derived from cells of widely different species. When fusion takes place between a normal cell and a cell from a malignant tumour, the daughter cells generally remain normal; but when in the course of several generations a considerable number of chromosomes have been eliminated the cells become malignant. This is probably due to the elimination of certain chromosomes rather than to a reduction in the total number of chromosomes (Harris 1971).

It has been shown (see page 39), that Driesch, by pressing early cleavage stages, contradicted Weismann's hypothesis of qualitatively different nuclear divisions as the basis for differentiation. That the nuclei keep all their potencies in the course of development has now been clearly demonstrated by the transplanting of amphibian nuclei from different tissues back into enucleated eggs to start the development over again (Briggs and King 1952, King and Briggs 1956, Gurdon 1968). However, what determines differentiation?—the main question of this book. In spite of his fundamental results on chromosomes, Boveri did not neglect the cytoplasm: in papers published in 1910, he showed that the chromatin diminution in *Ascaris* eggs is released by the cytoplasm. Already, in his famous paper (1901*b*), he had stated that only an animal–vegetal stratification can explain the larval differentiation of the sea-urchin embryo. Morgan, who in his early days belonged to the sea-urchin experimental embryologists in Naples, has elaborated the theory of nucleo-cytoplasmic interactions (1934, p. 234). He considers that the basic constitution of the gene remains always the same but that they are changing in some way, as development proceeds, in response to that part of the cytoplasm in which they come to lie, and these changes have a reciprocal influence on the cytoplasm. In modern wording the nuclei are equipotential; most genes at the beginning of the development being dormant (depressed) but, by and by, activated (redepressed) under influence of the cytoplasm in the different parts of the embryo, including gradual changes of the cytoplasm because of further interactions with the nuclei.

Boveri also raised the question whether the chromosomes alone are responsible for all transfer of inherited characters. To attack this problem he invented the method of experiments with merogones. Loeb (1899) had showed that eggs activated to parthenogenesis could produce normal larvae although their chromosome set is only haploid. Boveri wanted to obtain sea-urchin eggs deprived of nucleus, fertilize them with spermatozoa of the same or another species (homosperm or heterosperm merogony) in order to obtain direct comparison of nuclear–cytoplasmic inheritance. Several papers are devoted to those experiments which, however, could not provide definitive results because the requisite technique was still lacking.

The first attempt to produce an organism with nucleus from one species and cytoplasm from another was made by Rauber (1886) in order to test the possible hereditary effect of cytoplasm. He removed the nucleus of a frog's egg by means of a pipette and injected it into a toad's egg which had also been deprived of his nucleus, but without result. The term merogony was coined by Delage in 1899. In 1889 Boveri isolated fragments of sea-urchin eggs by violent shaking. Such fragments, after homosperm fertilization, could develop into plutei. As hybrid plutei of *Sphaerechinus granularis* ♀ × *Psammechinus microtuberculatus* ♂ were obtained with intermediate skeletal characters, he started merogony experiments with this combination. In cultures with a great number of fragments he found intermediate and paternal plutei and concluded that the latter emanated from egg fragments without egg nuclei. This statement created a sensation but also aroused much opposition. Hybrids vary considerably and even may have a paternal skeleton (Seeliger 1894, 1896, Morgan 1895e, Steinbruck 1902); their appearance can vary with the season and the degree of maturity of the gametes (Vernon 1900; Koehler 1914, 1916). Herbst (1906a) drew attention to the influence of the temperature. A clear picture was given in a posthumous paper by Boveri (1918): real heterosperm merogones of the combination referred to can develop only as far as the onset of gastrulation; shaking can break the nucleus in different ways into invisible pieces, or it may even happen that the whole nucleus escapes detection after bursting of the membrane. On the other hand, Boveri believed that the size of the nuclei could settle the question whether merogony was present or not. However, this statement is also doubtful as regards the variability of nuclear size.

In a paper published in 1914(a), Boveri described dwarf plutei of the combination *Psammechinus* cytoplasm + *Paracentrotus* nucleus as true merogones. However, in this case also the origin of the larvae remains uncertain. He added that this combination in any case provided no answer as to the localization of heredity factors, since he found no different species characters in the plutei.

The glass needle technique has provided the weapon with which to attack the merogony problem anew by dividing a mature unfertilized egg into a fragment containing the nucleus (n), and a cytoplasmic (cpl) part (Hörstadius 1936c). As the nucleus has an eccentric position the nucleated fragment can be made rather small (Fig. 71). Its exact position in relation to the egg axis cannot be identified, but the removal of this small amount of cytoplasm will not prevent development to pluteus, as shown in Chapter 6.

The first step was to find combinations allowing not only development but also differentiation of reliable species characters. It is striking that many combinations form hybrid plutei, often with clear intermediate characters, whereas their merogones show poor development, if any. Taylor and Tennent (1924) fertilized 49 egg fragments of *Toxopneustes* with *Tripneustes* sperm: only 15 started segmentation and only one reached blastula stage. Fry (1927) obtained only 46 blastulae from 869 merogones *Echinarachnius* cpl + *Arbacia* n. Ethel Brown Harvey (1933)

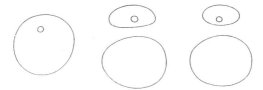

FIG. 71. The nucleus together with a small part of the cytoplasm is removed with a glass needle from the greater part of a mature egg. (From Hörstadius 1936c.)

reported plutei of *Sphaerechinus* cpl + *Paracentrotus* n, the fragments obtained by centrifugation. In my paper in 1936(c) (p. 813) I expressed strong doubts as to the validity of the technique and its results. In his extensive paper of 1954, von Ubisch in co-operation with E. B. Harvey has repeated the work with centrifugation and states that the method is not suited for merogony experiments. When I repeated these experiments I found that the species used by Boveri confirmed his results. Cytoplasm of *Paracentrotus lividus* or *Psammechinus microtuberculatus* fertilized with *Sphaerechinus* sperm gave only young blastulae. The reciprocal combinations could lead to gastrulae and in some cases to prism-shaped larvae, which, however, had poor archenteron and skeleton. Some of the egg fragments did not even commence development. The combination of these species was particularly desirable as the fenestrated rods of *Sphaerechinus* provide definite species characters compared to the single smooth rods of the other species (see below). von Ubisch (1959) has also tried merogones with *Genocidaris maculata* as one of the components. *Psammechinus microtuberculatus* cpl + *Genocidaris* n died as blastulae. In the reciprocal combination 143 died as blastulae and only 8 reached the gastrula stage. Of *Genocidaris* cpl + *Paracentrotus* n, a few went as far as to prism or young pluteus stages but they were too abnormal to allow interpretation of species characters to be made.

Shearer, de Morgan, and Fuchs (1914) succeeded in rearing hybrids of *Echinus esculentus* and *Psammechinus miliaris* through metamorphosis to full-grown sea-urchins. Although I myself in Plymouth also brought hybrid larvae to metamorphosis and homosperm merogones formed plutei, the merogones *Psammechinus* cpl. + *Echinus* n did not reach further than to the blastula stage. The best result with the reciprocal combination was two gastrulae with a diminutive archenteron and small triradiate spicules. These larvae thus did not in differentiation surpass those with *Sphaerechinus* as one of the components. No doubt the most suitable combination for merogony experiments as regards viability is *Psammechinus microtuberculatus* with *Paracentrotus lividus* (Naples). The same favourable outcome might be expected from combining *Paracentrotus* with another very similar *Psammechinus*, namely *miliaris* (Roscoff); but experiments showed the contrary. Not even hybrids were attained with eggs of *Paracentrotus*. Neither eggs nor fragments without nuclei could be activated by *Psammechinus miliaris* sperm. On the other hand, a few larvae of *Psammechinus miliaris* cpl + *Paracentrotus* n got as far as young but irregular plutei (1936c, Abb. 2).

On the basis of his experiments with merogony and dispermic eggs, Boveri (1918) advanced the hypothesis that we are dealing with two essentially different periods in early development as regards participation of the nucleus. In the first period, the constitution of the cytoplasm should be decisive, while only some general qualities of the nucleus are requisite. In the second period, the specific qualities of the chromosomes should assert themselves. In their absence the larva is doomed. A heterosperm merogone cannot develop further than to early gastrulation as the foreign chromosomes do not co-operate with the cytoplasm. In disperm larvae the chromosomes cannot function properly as they are not present in the right combination. In hybrids the set of maternal chromosomes is enough to ensure the normal course of necessary metabolic processes, while the sperm chromosomes can contribute to species characters.

On the basis of observations on somatic 'cell hybrids' (see p. 136) Ephrussi and colleagues (Siniscalco 1969) have suggested the classification of biochemical functions of somatic cells into 'essential' and 'luxury' functions. The former should include the metabolic processes which are necessary to keep the life of the cell going, while the luxury functions should act in service of the individual as a whole. This notion seems to have a certain resemblance to Boveri's hypothesis. The term 'luxury' is perhaps not a good choice. Processes which build tissue and act within tissues and organs are indispensable for the life of the organism and are in no sense a luxury. In contrast to those functions which are imperative for the life of the cell, the other functions could be characterized as 'specialized'. If the differentiation also leads to physiological differences in relation to other species the cells are also 'speciesized'.

The Boveri's hypothesis has been supported by modern investigations concerning the moment of onset of genic action (Barros, Hand, jr., and Monroy 1966; Ebert and Sussex 1970; Giudice, Mutolo, and Donatuti 1968; Glisin and Glisin 1964; Westin 1969). The early development through cleavage is considered to depend mainly on the action of the maternal genes, large amounts of nucleic acids having been synthesized during oogenesis. Unfertilized eggs are said to contain a complete 'programme' for early development, up to the onset of gastrulation, in the form of cytoplasmically-stored templates. Most protein is thus encoded by maternal RNA. New synthesis of RNAs in sea-urchin begins after fertilization, the quantity doubling in connexion with the cell divisions. However, the embryonic genes are genetically more or less 'silent' until, at varying times after fertilization depending on the species, they are activated and new RNAs are formed—which is evidence of the sequential activation of the genome in sea-urchins. The normal rate of protein synthesis in oocytes and eggs of *Xenopus laevis* was found to be limited by their content of functional messenger RNA, as injected messenger RNA disclosed an unused capacity for translation (Moar *et al.* 1971). The genic action becomes particularly intense at the beginning of sea-urchin gastrulation, which requires new production of templates. It is at this point that the biparental origin of the zygote becomes manifest.

However, other facts do not comply with the notion of a late start of nuclear activity. We have seen on p. 81 that eggs can be divided into two halves by centrifugation in a density gradient. The plane of division is arbitrary in relation to the egg axis. The anucleated 'red halves' can give plutei after fertilization. Harvey (1936) also found that such halves could be activated parthenogenetically. Centrosomes become replicated, asters are formed and eggs divide into a number of 'cells' without nuclei. Unfertilized sea-urchin eggs synthesize very little protein, but fertilization induces a rapid increase in protein synthesis (Monroy 1965). A similar increase starts also after parthenogenetic activation of anucleate fragments. They evidently possess the information necessary for cleavage and protein synthesis (Brachet *et al.* 1963). The cleavage is not normal, however, and the most successful cases only lead to a morula, perhaps with a cavity. The 'cells' cannot differentiate, they remain as spheroidal cleavage cells incapable of forming a blastula wall with cylindric ciliated epithelium. They are therefore unable to reach the stage of beginning gastrulation, when the genes of the zygot have been found to take charge of protein synthesis. Furthermore, it seems dubious whether DNA synthesis is possible in the absence of a nucleus. (Lit. in reviews by Brachet 1970, 1971a, b).

Nor do some observations concerning hybrids and merogones support the hypothesis that the paternal genes hardly come into action before gastrulation. Reciprocal hybridizations sometimes show differences in viability. As the pairs of nuclei are the same, the difference must be due to the cytoplasm. In the heterosperm merogony experiments, reported here at some length in order to serve as material for this discussion, it was stated, for example, that the sperm could not activate an egg fragment, while the reciprocal combination could lead to young, although irregular, plutei. According to viability a series of different combinations extends from death at cleavage stages or as young or old blastulae, early gastrulae, prism stages or young plutei up to healthy plutei capable of feeding and further differentiation. It is noteworthy that frequently only a few specimens reached blastula or abnormal gastrula stage, whereas the majority succumbed during cleavage. While von Ubisch (1959) went much further than Boveri in stating that in hybrids the genetic differences first become injurious in the pluteus stage it seems that the merogone results point towards cleavage as the critical period in several combinations. Homosperm merogones do excellently. In spite of the presumed maternal programme, a foreign nucleus may be the cause of poor development because of its incapacity to transcribe some substances that are necessary in early stages. For another example of early nuclear activity see page 172.

The reasons for the impossibility of co-operation between cytoplasm and alien nucleus have been studied in lethal hybrid combinations of the species *Paracentrotus lividus* (*PP*), *Arbacia lixula* (*AA*), and *Sphaerechinus granularis* (*SS*). In the hybrids *PS* (*P*♀ × *S*♂) paternal chromosomes were already eliminated during the first cleavage, and the larvae hardly reached an inhibited gastrula stage. In the hybrids *PA* and *AP* no chromatin elimination could be detected, but the reduced volume of nuclei in aged embryos possibly indicates elimination between blastula and gastrula stages. These hybrids died at a somewhat more advanced gastrula stage because of pyknosis of the nuclei. (Baltzer 1910; Baltzer and Chen 1960, 1965; Baltzer *et al.* 1961.)

In larvae of pure species the amount of DNA was found, by isotopic labelling, to increase in the course of development, while the RNA remained almost constant. In *PA*, *AP*, *PS*, and *SP*, the DNA synthesis was intermediate to or lower than that in the parent species, but DNA inhibition had no effect on total RNA which remained normal in the hybrids. These, however, showed a definite reduction in RNA turnover and DNA synthesis. The decrease of DNA synthesis in hybrids was found to parallel the decrease in the number of nuclei, and—an essential point—both processes were parallel to the morphogenetic inhibitions. It was an open question which of these three factors was the primary one. Amphibian merogones *Triton palmatus* cpl $+$ *Triton cristatus* n showed a marked drop in the amount of both DNA and RNA during neurulation, before death, owing to cell degeneration at later stages. (Baltzer *et al.* 1961; Chen and Baltzer 1962, 1964; Baltzer and Chen 1965.)

By studying the total uptake of ^{3}H-thymidine per embryo, the total number of nuclei, and the percentage of radioactive nuclei, Baltzer *et al.* (1967) found that *PP* had twice as high DNA synthesis per nucleus as *AA*. The difference is tentatively explained by the much greater length of *PP* chromosomes. In blastulae with mesenchyme cells the *PA* hybrids incorporated less than *PP* and *AA*, while at the gastrula stage the values for *PA* were intermediate. Diametrically opposed, however, are the observations by Ficq and Brachet (1963), who used autoradiographic methods. *AA* nuclei incorporated twice as much as those of *PP*, and for *PA* the values were higher than those for *PP* and *AA*.

Applying the technique of molecular hybridization, Denis and Brachet (1969*a*, *b*) stated that *PA* hybrids contain about 2·5 times as much *P* DNA as DNA of paternal origin. Labelled *PP* and *AA* RNA hybridized about 2·5 times better with DNA of their own species than with DNA of the other species. However, RNA from *PA* hybridized about twice as well with paternal *AA* DNA as with maternal *PP* DNA although the hybrids contain more maternal than paternal DNA. Further investigations suggested the following interpretation of this surprising result (Denis and Brachet 1970). Transcription of the genome was found to be partially stage-specific, since in pure species embryos, RNA from unfertilized eggs and from plutei is less competitive against labelled RNA from gastrulae than gastrula RNA itself. This stage-specificity is maintained in the hybrid as far as transcription of the maternal genome is concerned, but is lost regarding the paternal genome. The *PA* gastrula synthesizes more RNA molecules of *AA* type than does the normal *AA* gastrula, whereas *PP* RNA is produced in equal amounts in *PP* and

PA embryos. These observations characterize the hybridization properties of the RNA synthesized by the blocked gastrula. The authors
suggest the occurrence of two kinds of genes. The one type transcribed
at all stages of development should be more active in foreign than in
their own cytoplasm, while genes with activity restricted to the gastrula
stage should not be able to function in foreign cytoplasm.

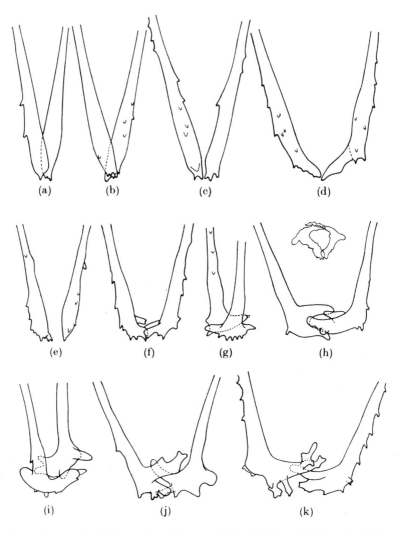

FIG. 72. (a)–(d) Body-rods of *Paracentrotus lividus*, (a)–(c) of plutei
20–21 days old, (d) 27 days old. (e)–(k) Body-rods of *Psammechinus
microtuberculatus*, (e) at age 4 days, (f), (g) 5 days, (h)–(j) 8 days, (k) 25 days.
(From Hörstadius 1936c.)

Larvae with foreign nuclei

The young plutei of both *Paracentrotus lividus* and *Psammechinus microtuberculatus* have single smooth arm-rods and body-rods. To begin with they show no distinguishing species characters; after five days, however, the body-rods of *Psammechinus* develop thickened irregular ends, bending towards each other, often forked and from both sides passing the median plane (Fig. 72(e)–(k)). The body-rods of *Paracentrotus* keep their straight, smooth form (a)–(c) although in some plutei after three or four weeks they may grow slightly towards each other (d) but without thickening and not in the same conspicuous way as in *Psammechinus*. Hybrids show intermediate types.

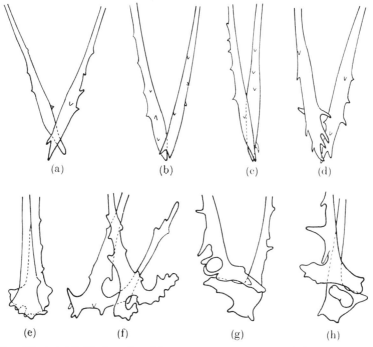

Fig. 73. (a)–(d) Body-rods of homosperm merogones of *Paracentrotus lividus*, 7–9 days old; (e)–(h) of *Psammechinus microtuberculatus*, 8–13 days old. (From Hörstadius 1936c.)

Homosperm merogones of both species differentiated in the expected way, with straight and irregular clubs (Fig. 73). In some larvae, however, there was a tendency towards overproduction, as discussed in following sections. The field was then open for experiments with heterosperm merogones. About 400 enucleated fragments of both species were fertilized. Many died at different stages or showed relatively poor development, but about 20 were able to swim and feed for weeks. In the merogones with *Psammechinus* nucleus, the body-rods reached the typical *Psammechinus* type with heavy irregular clubs (Fig. 74(c), (d), Fig. 75(j)–(o)), the first case of a paternal character developed in an animal organism with cytoplasm of one species and nucleus of another. In the reciprocal combination, with *Paracentrotus* nuclei, the result was somewhat puzzling. It is true that the rods on the whole developed as expected, slender and straight (Fig. 74(a), (b), Fig. 75(a)–(e)). Some, however, developed atypical protuberances, but they were not broad and

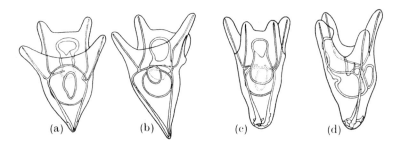

FIG. 74. (a), (b) Heterosperm merogones of *Psammechinus* cytoplasm +
Paracentrotus nucleus, 12 and 9 days old. (c), (d) *Paracentrotus* cytoplasm
+ *Psammechinus* nucleus, 8 and 11 days old. (From Hörstadius 1936c.)

massive, nor so markedly bent towards each other as in the *Psamme-chinus* rods (Fig. 75(f)–(i)). Most of them protruded a little way from the end of the rod, thus not constituting a thickening of the extreme terminal part, as in *Psammechinus*, and they could grow as slender branches parallel to the body-rod. They did not resemble the clubs of *Psamm-echinus*, nor were they similar to the body-rods of three- to four-weeks-old *Paracentrotus* plutei, in which the terminal parts rarely can grow towards each other although without thickening (Fig. 72(d)).

In the heterosperm merogones with *Psammechinus* nucleus (Fig. 75 (j)–(o)) the differentiation according to the nucleus was clearly established. A possible plasmatic effect is not discernible. However, how can the deviations from the smooth type in the reciprocal combination be interpreted? Are they to be attributed to plasmatic inheritance, or are other factors involved? Several experiments were made to elucidate this problem.

As temperature has been found to affect differentiation in hybrids (see page 138) larvae of *Paracentrotus lividus* at Roscoff (sea temperature

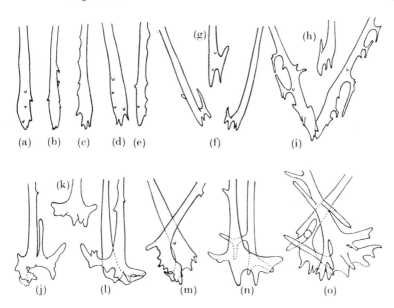

FIG. 75. (a–i) Body-rods of heterosperm merogones *Psammechinus* cytoplasm + *Paracentrotus* nucleus 9–12 days old; (j–o) of *Paracentrotus* cytoplasm + *Psammechinus* nucleus 8–11 days old. (From Hörstadius 1936c.)

16°–18°C) were reared at 28°C. It is known that cleavage stages are particularly sensitive to high temperature (Hörstadius 1925d). The larvae therefore were placed in the thermostat as swimming blastulae. While hundreds of plutei remained normal some were found to develop irregular thickening of the body-rods (Fig. 76(a)–(d)), some of them (c) more resembling *Psammechinus* rods than the irregularities in our merogones. von Ubisch (1932b) and Nümann (1933) showed that warmth may lead to excessive calcification.

It has been stated that left and right halves of *Paracentrotus* isolated at the onset of gastrulation have skeleton only on the non-operated side, but that they start to regenerate missing parts and also coelom (see Chapters 7 and 8). In such halves the body-rods could present outgrowths towards the defective side which also resembled those in the merogones but were even further developed (Fig. 76(e)–(g)). Moreover, body-rods of the divergent form under discussion were found in plutei of hybrids (both combinations), in homosperm *Psammechinus* merogones, and in heterosperm merogones with *Psammechinus* nucleus, thus in larvae with haploid *Psammechinus* chromosomes (1936c, Abb. 24, 25).

A comparison between the clubs of *Psammechinus* control plutei, on the one hand (Fig. 72(e)–(k)), and both homosperm and heterosperm merogones with *Psammechinus* nuclei, on the other hand (Fig. 73(e–h), Fig. 75(j)–(o)), in some cases gives the impression of excessive development of the clubs in the latter two groups, as regards volume and irregular shape. The constitution of our merogones is not ideal initially because the cytoplasm is too large in relation to the haploid nucleus, and, in addition, part of the cytoplasm has been removed, causing a certain

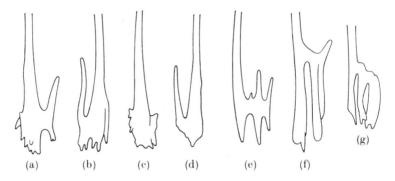

FIG. 76. (a)–(d) Body-rods of *Paracentrotus lividus* plutei, 4–5 days old, reared at Roscoff at 28 °C (sea temperature 16–18 °C). (e)–(g) Body-rods of meridional half plutei, isolated at beginning gastrulation, 4–7 days old. (From Hörstadius 1936c.)

imbalance in the gradient system. There is no doubt that the *Psammechinus* character is introduced by the sperm. In heterosperm merogones it may attain a typical and even exaggerated form; when present only in haploid state, however, it does not always attain typical shape but instead resembles the *Paracentrotus* rods, with atypical outgrowths.

Are these atypical protrusions in the reciprocal heterosperm combination, with *Paracentrotus* nucleus, due to *Psammechinus* cytoplasmic inheritance? The fact that rods of this shape can be found in the presence of haploid *Psammechinus* nuclei could lead us to consider them as a weak *Psammechinus* character. Against this interpretation must be put forward certain observations concerning similar differentiations occurring at raised temperature (Fig. 76(a)–(d)), and in halves as attempted regeneration (e)–(g). The atypical *Paracentrotus* outgrowths, never seen in control cultures nor in homosperm merogones, represent a skeletal overproduction perhaps comparable to the excessive growth of clubs in some homosperm and heterosperm merogones with *Psammechinus* nuclei (Fig. 73(e)–(h)), Fig. 75(j)–(o)). Too high a temperature is an unfavourable environmental factor. Possibly cytoplasm from another species, in conjunction with the altered quantitative relationships referred to above, constitute unfavourable conditions for the nucleus and result in increased calcification.

von Ubisch (1957) has repeated the merogony experiments with the same species. His observations on the whole confirm those mentioned above. In old *Paracentrotus* plutei he did not find any body-rods bent like those in Fig. 72(d). They were all of the straight type, thus not at all resembling *Psammechinus* clubs. On the other hand, he described homosperm *Psammechinus* merogones which have a still more complex structure of the clubs than shown in Fig. 73(e)–(h), and thus provide another example of overproduction in a haploid larva. In merogones with *Paracentrotus* nuclei he also found cases with aberrations more exaggerated than in Fig. 75(f)–(i). In spite of this he rejected the possibility of cytoplasmic inheritance. He found the heavy, distal, median-directed clubs of *Psammechinus* essentially different from the slender projections in *Paracentrotus*, often parallel to the body-rod. He is in no case in doubt as to which species the nucleus in a larva belongs, concurring in the idea that in larvae with *Paracentrotus* nucleus can high temperature, fragmentation, and haploid state as modifying factors promote excessive skeletal growth.

In spite of the unfavourable previous reports, von Ubisch (1954) used eggs of *Sphaerechinus granularis* and sperm of *Paracentrotus* or *Psamme-chinus microtuberculatus* for merogony experiments at Naples. With sperm of *Paracentrotus* and egg fragments from the third batch he obtained two young plutei. The subsequent results were unsuccessful until the 80th batch, with *Psammechinus* sperm, when he found 14 plutei which were reared and drawn between the ages of 3 and 45 days. To reach this result he fertilized about 3000 fragments.

One of the best merogones is reproduced in Fig. 77. The skeleton in the larva was paternal, with no attempts made to form the fenestrated rods which are characteristic of *Sphaerechinus*. However, the ends of the body-rods developed pointed outgrowths in different directions (Scheitel-strahlen) of a type unfamiliar to both species. This is reminiscent of the excessive growth of the body-rod clubs in the *Paracentrotus* + *Psamme-chinus* and *Psammechinus* + *Paracentrotus* merogones. Only anterior ciliary epaulettes which are typical of the male parent were formed. There were no signs of *Sphaerechinus* posterior epaulettes and lobes; von Ubisch therefore stated that the external form at first sight was entirely paternal, but that the maternal body form became more and more apparent, the apex growing more rounded. It seems doubtful to me that this was a proof of plasmatic inheritance. von Ubisch ascribed the outgrowth of the 'Scheitelstrahlen' to a stretching of the mesenchymal skeleton-forming syncytium (not directly observed) because of the widening of the ectoderm. This explanation should apply also to the overproduction observed in the experiments described earlier. The direction of the body-rods may vary under experimental conditions; when the angle between them is broader than normally, the body-wall

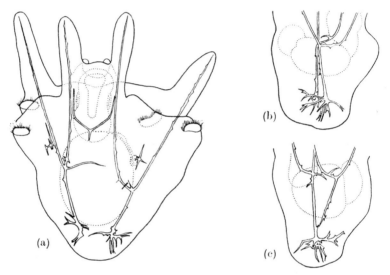

FIG. 77. Heterosperm merogones *Sphaerechinus granularis* cytoplasm + *Psammechinus microtuberculatus* nucleus (a) 35, (b) 18, and (c) 29 days old. (From von Ubisch 1954.)

also widens, without mechanical contact. It is impossible to determine whether the overproduction in the first place depends upon action from the ectoderm.

von Ubisch was well aware of the strange fact that a satisfactory development occurred only within two batches and gave no more than 14 plutei of about 3000 merogones. This could indicate the presence of some special conditions—for example, invisible partial nuclei. von Ubisch worked very cautiously and critically. The number of chromosomes in merogones was found to be haploid. The nuclear dimensions in merogone plutei were smaller than those found in the paternal diploid form; the nuclei, however, were larger than the haploid nuclei. The hypothesis was put forward that the nuclei of *Psammechinus* and

Paracentrotus under the influence of the *Sphaerechinus* cytoplasm attained the size corresponding to the latter species. von Ubisch discussed the results with an eye to two alternatives: that the plutei were pure merogones, or larvae which, besides paternal chromatin, also contained a limited quantity of maternal chromatin derived from nuclear fragments. In both cases it was clear that the skeletal pattern, without any trace of fenestrated rods, as well as the relative length of the larval arms, the epaulettes, and the posterior lobes, were due to the nuclei. In my opinion the shape of the body, particularly with regard to the atypical body-rods, is hardly a character distinctive enough to prove plasmatic inheritance.

10 *Germ-layer chimeras*

CHIMERAS are organisms in which one part of the body or some tissues belong to one species, while the other part belongs to another species. The production of organisms consisting of germ-layers from different species is of interest for the study of interactions between tissues and organs with genetic differences.

Baltzer (1920–35) studied amphibian merogones. The *Triton* egg often receives several sperms (physiological polyspermy). Baltzer obtained heterosperm merogones by isolation (constriction method of Spemann) of half-eggs devoid of egg nucleus but containing sperm of another species. At a certain stage, different for different species combinations, the larvae died because the nuclei of the head mesenchyme became diseased. Baltzer (1930) and Hadorn (1930–37) then adopted the chimera principle by transplanting pieces of merogones into normal larvae, where they could develop further. The epidermis and muscles, in particular, proved viable. However, no tissues differentiated so far as to show species character of the nucleus. Instead transplanted merogone epidermis with nuclei from a species with smooth skin and cytoplasm from a species with rough skin after metamorphosis had obtained an epidermis of the rough type. Apparently only hosts with rough skin were used. As it was shown that a normal host can stimulate lethal hybrid tissues to viability the possibility may exist of an host influence also on the differentiation of the skin in the course of the development through metamorphosis.

When beginning the sea-urchin merogone experiments my intention was to use germ-layer chimeras if a tissue of heterosperm merogones did not develop in a healthy way. Because of the high viability of the merogones the plan was not made use of for that purpose; nevertheless, it may be of interest to mention some chimera experiments. Bierens de Haan (1913*a*, *b*) succeeded in fusing fragments of normal larvae of *Psammechinus microtuberculatus* and *Paracentrotus lividus*. However, as the fusion occurred at random, no integrated plutei were formed, and as no fusion succeeded between the less related *Psammechinus* or *Paracentrotus* on the one hand, and *Sphaerechinus granularis* and *Arbacia lixula* on the other, no conclusion could be drawn as to interaction on species characters. von Ubisch (1931) tried transplantation at cleavage stages, but without success. However, heteroplastic fusions with the desired orientation can be made with the transplantation method shown in Fig. 9 if the pressure by the small glass ball is continued for several hours (Hörstadius 1936*c*). Meridional halves of *Paracentrotus* and *Psammechinus* brought together could give rise to plutei, but in such larvae a possible influence of ectoderm on the differentiation of the clubs could not be studied, as the primary mesenchyme cells might be mixed.

von Ubisch used another method to study such interrelations. In a number of papers between 1931 and 1939 (lit. in 1939) he described the result of implanting micromeres of one species into the blastocoele of another. Unfortunately, the age of the blastulae used was never indicated. In order to obtain pure germ-layer chimeras he implanted micromeres into blastulae from animal halves isolated at cleavage stages $(8+0+0)$ or from entire presumptive ectoderm $(8+veg_1+0)$. However, as the blastulae at the implantation were too old to react to the inductive force of the micromeres (cf. Fig. 40) they were unable, in the absence of digestive tract and arms, to form any typical skeleton. von Ubisch also implanted micromeres into whole blastulae. The larvae then contained two sets of skeleton-forming cells. If the one species had plain skeletal rods, such as *Psammechinus* (Fig. 78(a)), and the other fenestrated rods, such as *Echinocardium* (b), the result was all kinds of intermediate types (c), (d). It seems unclear whether the mixture of different structures was due to a mosaic of the mesenchyme cells of the two species, or to the formation of a mixed syncytium. The role of the ectoderm for the outgrowth of long rods was illustrated by the fact that an unpaired body-rod, as in the plutei of *Echinocardium*, appeared only in a chimera with ectoderm of that species (d).

Complete chimeras were obtained by fusing the presumptive ectoderm $(8+veg_1+0)$ of *Psammechinus microtuberculatus* with the presumptive endomesoderm (veg_2+4) of *Paracentrotus lividus* (Fig. 79(a), (b)).

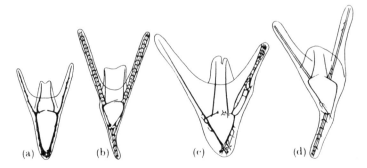

FIG. 78. Experiments with germ-layer chimeras. The digestive tracts
were omitted in the original drawings. (a) Pluteus of *Psammechinus microtuberculatus*. (b) Pluteus of *Echinocardium cordatum*. (c) Chimera of whole
blastula of *Psammechinus* + micromeres of *Echinocardium*. (d) Whole
blastula of *Echinocardium* + micromeres of *Psammechinus*. The skeleton
is mixed in both chimeras because of presence of primary mesenchyme
of both species. (From von Ubisch 1934.)

Since the body-rods were of *Paracentrotus* type, there was no sign of
influence from the *Psammechinus* ectoderm.

A subsequent step was an attempt to obtain chimera plutei by implanting micromeres into animal halves or $8 + veg_1 + 0$. In contrast
to the experiments of von Ubisch, the implantation should be performed

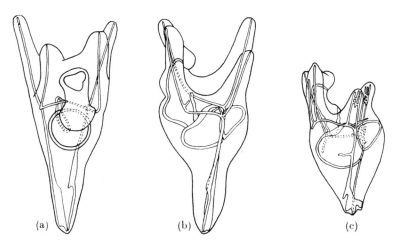

FIG. 79. (a, b) Presumptive ectoderm $(8 + veg_1)$ from *Psammechinus* +
presumptive endo- and mesoderm $(veg_2 + 4)$ from *Paracentrotus*. (c) $8 +
veg_1$ of *Psammechinus* + 4 micromeres of *Sphaerechinus granularis*.
Fenestrated anal rods and ramified ends of body-rods are *Sphaerechinus*
characters. (From Hörstadius 1936*c*.)

at an early cleavage stage in order to give the chimera chance of induction between cells of different species. It has been shown that for heteroplastic transplantation a much-prolonged pressure was necessary for fusion. Then another difficulty arose. Fig. 30 illustrates the remarkable faculty of an animal half to seize and eject a piece of cytoplasm without nucleus, which evidently is interpreted as a foreign and undesirable body. Another method was also used to reject such a piece, namely, by making an opening between the blastomeres through which it could fall out. In combinations of micromeres and halves from more closely related species, such as *Psammechinus*, *Paracentrotus*, and *Sphaerechinus*, the implantation could be performed in the customary way. However, in experiments with species from different orders, the regular *Sphaerechinus granularis* and the irregular *Echinocardium cordatum*, both of these strange methods came into use. In all the 20 cases, including both combinations, the micromeres were ejected within one or two hours. The micromeres were replaced in one of the halves which, after the ejection, still had the shape of a bowl; after a while they were ejected for the second time. It is almost incredible that animal halves of the intellectual level of blastomeres, first, are able to distinguish as undesirable both cytoplasm without nucleus and micromeres from a distantly related species (in contrast to closer relatives), and secondly, have two methods of getting rid of them. The ejection could, in some cases, be avoided by using $8+veg_1+0$ instead of halves, as these fragments have a smaller opening. Induction of archenteron took place only in the combination with *Echinocardium* micromeres in *Paracentrotus* ectoderm, but the development of the skeleton was poor. This result was sufficient to show that the inductive capacity of micromeres could assert itself also in presumptive ectoderm that was not closely related.

Psammechinus and *Sphaerechinus* belong to different families of the regular sea-urchins. A pluteus was obtained after implantation of *Sphaerechinus* micromeres into the entire presumptive ectoderm of *Psammechinus microtuberculatus* (Fig. 79(c)). Induction thus led to the formation of a typical alimentary canal. Fenestrated anal rods, ramified ends of body-rods, and rudiments of posterior body-rods are *Sphaerechinus* characters.

Germ-layer chimeras have also been made with blastomeres of a heterosperm merogone forming one fragment. The idea was to give the nuclei of the skeleton-forming cells of one species the chance of developing the species character without any possible participation by their own cytoplasm. The micromeres from a merogone *Paracentrotus* cpl with *Psammechinus* nuclei (Fig. 80(a)$_1$) were isolated. In order to avoid mixing of primary mesenchyme cells from host and donor they were implanted not into a whole egg but into the presumptive ectoderm of *Paracentrotus* (a)$_2$, (a)$_3$. The implantation offered no difficulty. There was no attempt at expulsion, the cytoplasm of both partners belonging to the same species and the nuclei to closely-related species. As a result, the new organism consisted of cytoplasm and nuclei of *Paracentrotus* with the

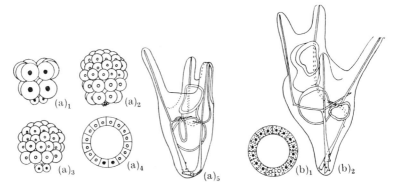

FIG. 80. (a)$_1$ Diagram of a 16-cell stage of a heterosperm merogone *Paracentrotus lividus* cytoplasm (white) + *Psammechinus microtuberculatus* nucleus (black). (a)$_2$ A 64-cell stage of *Paracentrotus* (nuclei white). (a)$_3$ The presumptive ectoderm (8+veg_1) of *Paracentrotus* combined with the micromeres of a merogone. (a)$_4$ The blastula consists of *Paracentrotus* cytoplasm and nuclei, except for the nuclei of the micromeres which equal the presumptive skeleton-forming cells. (a)$_5$ These nuclei give the pluteus the appearance of a *Psammechinus* larva (the thickened, bent, irregular clubs of the body-rods). (b)$_1$ The reciprocal combination. (b)$_2$ Although the larva consists of *Psammechinus* cytoplasm (dotted in (b)$_1$) and nuclei (except the nuclei of the skeleton-forming cells), the pluteus looks like a *Paracentrotus* larva (straight, slender body-rods). (From Hörstadius 1936*c*.)

exception of the nuclei in the descendants of the micromeres (a)$_4$. Any expert on plutei of these species would designate the larva (a)$_5$ as a *Psammechinus* pluteus, the clubs of the body-rods having attained the typical species character. That the nuclei alone were the carriers of this character cannot be called into question as no cytoplasm of *Psammechinus* was present.

The reciprocal combination (b)$_1$, (b)$_2$ confirmed the result. The body-rods were of the straight slender *Paracentrotus* type, although the cytoplasm of the skeleton-forming cells belonged to the species with heavy irregular clubs. Nor was the *Psammechinus* ectoderm able to exert an influence on the body-rods in a *Psammechinus* direction.

On review of the results reported in chapters 9 and 10 there seem to be no doubt that it has been possible to prove by a direct experiment that a nucleus of one species in the cytoplasm of another is able to bring forth a positive species character, where the one species has a more complex skeletal structure than the other. The suspicion could arise that the irregular clubs of *Psammechinus* are dependent on the influence of the ectoderm, as the growth of arm rods and arm ectoderm is a result of mutual interactions. However, the clubs appeared also in chimeras with pure *Paracentrotus* ectoderm. There no material outside the primary mesenchyme nuclei was a carrier of *Psammechinus* faculties (Fig. 80(a)). In contrast, in the reciprocal chimera combination neither the *Psammechinus* cytoplasm in the skeleton-forming cells nor the pure *Psammechinus* ectoderm was able to entice the differentiation into a *Psammechinus* direction.

The experiments have not supported the hypothesis of the occurrence of cytoplasmic inheritance. The aberrations described in *Paracentrotus* rods did not have a real *Psammechinus* character. Possible explanations were discussed. The only clear influence of cytoplasm was on the size of the larvae, larger plutei emanating from larger eggs. This, however, is a quantitative matter without genetic significance in the sense dealt with here, the egg size depending on the nuclei and maternal conditions.

11 *Some aspects of determination*

BOVERI expressed as early as 1901(*b*) the hypothesis that the first differentiation begins more easily at one point than at all others. 'If the differentiation has started here, then all other regions will have their role determined by regulation emanating from that point' (translated from the German). In the first publications on transplantations in sea-urchin embryos, the inductive effect of the most vegetal material was interpreted as the action of an organizer (Hörstadius 1928). The results tallied with the demands of Spemann for a centre of organization. A stream of determination proceeded from the vegetal material, of which a piece, after implantation in indifferent (animal) material, could bring about development of a harmonious larva. Further investigations revealing the antagonistic forces of the animal material have, however, proved the immense advantage of applying the double gradient notion of Runnström.

In the egg the experimenter has to deal not only with the system along the egg axis, but also with the gradients along the ventro–dorsal and left–right axes. However, there is a difference in principle between the animal–vegetal axis and the other two. The properties of the animal and vegetal systems are very different, producing different organs: they are hostile, a strong predominance of the one leading to suppression of the other. A certain balance is required to attain harmonious development. After transverse sections the fragments, as a rule, exhibit the properties of both gradients; only in isolated micromeres and isolated an_1-cells do their own qualities completely prevail. However, or vegetal fragments or stretched eggs never display differentiations characteristic of the dominating pole also at the other end of the larva, with a kind of neutral region between them; there is no reversal of the axis in isolated fragments. In this respect the other two systems are notably different. Dorsal halves acquire a new ventral side on their most dorsal side—that is, after reversal of the ventro–dorsal axis (see Fig. 46). In embryos stretched perpendicular to the egg axis as well as in embryos partly divided by meridional constriction (see Fig. 47) ventral sides appear at both ends. The explanation has been given that all parts of the egg have an inherent capacity to form a ventral side (see Fig. 44) but that this capacity is normally inhibited by the presumptive ventral centre. Not even isolation is necessary to liberate the dorsal side from this inhibition; a prolonged distance has the same effect. Regulations within giants were interpreted in the same way (see Figs. 52, 53). The ventral centre can be subdued by chemical means. The result is larvae with radial symmetry (see Fig. 55).

As to the bilateral asymmetry, the starting point in several of the classes is a coelomic system with rudiments of anterior, middle, and posterior coeloms on both sides (see Fig. 57). Normally, the left middle coelom differentiates as a hydrocoele while the corresponding vesicle on the right side becomes reduced. However, in isolated right halves a hydrocoele may be found on the left or the right side or on both sides (Fig. 62(a)–(c)). The variations were attributed to relative strength of left and right tendencies in the form of gradients to produce a hydrocoele (d)–(f). The explanation could also be expressed in the same way as for the ventro–dorsal axis, an inhibition emanating from the left side in some halves being insufficiently strong to stop an inherent right potency from asserting itself. Here again it is a question not of qualitatively different forces but of the same kind of organ appearing at the opposite pole.

While both the ventral centre and the left side are trying to inhibit the development of an exact image of themselves at the other pole, an oral field, and a hydrocoele, the animal and vegetal systems, when properly strengthened, endeavour to subdue an adversary of a very different kind and to penetrate the body as much as possible along the axis.

In pure isolations and transplantations of animal and vegetal fragments, the effect was due to quantitative alterations of the animal–vegetal balance. The metabolic processes were not impeded from the outside. Lindahl (1936) obtained surprising results by animalizing eggs before fertilization by NaSCN in Ca-free sea-water (Fig. 81(a, b)) and, after fertilization, by vegetalizing them with lithium ions (c, d). The animalization did not spread gradually vegetal-wards but instead created a new animal centre at the presumptive vegetal pole (b). The lithium action followed this pattern, establishing endoderm between two ectodermal vesicles (c, d). The larva thus reversed the polarity of its vegetal part. Such larvae resemble larvae with the vegetal half reversed by transplantation (see Fig. 24). Lindahl explains the phenomenon as a case of 'polar dominance' similar to that observed in the ventro–dorsal axis. These results do not contradict my earlier statement on fundamental differences between animal and vegetal gradients, as they were the result of artificial encroachment on the metabolism by extrinsic animalizing and subsequent vegetalizing agents.

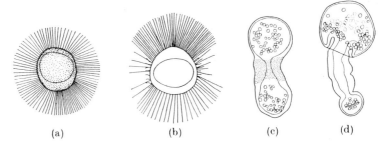

FIG. 81. (a, b) Whole eggs animalized after treatment with NaSCN before fertilization. (c, d) Reversal of the egg axis in the vegetal part of whole eggs after animalization by NaSCN before fertilization, and vegetalization by LiCl after fertilization. (Redrawn from Lindahl 1936.)

Child (1941, pp. 142, 240) was critical of the notion of two opposite, qualitatively different gradients. Local specific differences at the onset of development would mean complete predetermination. A single gradient of metabolic rate is considered to be the effective factor in development of organismal pattern. Although this idea would accord with changes in animalization or vegetalization with increasing concentration of agents, the hostility between animal and vegetal regions as well as many physiological results speak for qualitative differences. As an example may be mentioned the lack of sulphate which, according to Herbst (1904), leads to radialization or animalization of whole eggs. An analysis of the role of sulphate in embryonic differentiation (Runnström *et al.* 1964) showed that animal halves also became animalized while the vegetal halves instead became vegetalized in sulphate-free medium (Fig. 82). Similar results were obtained by rearing halves in a mixture of CO and CO_2 in darkness (Hörstadius and Strömberg 1940). Animal halves reared at low temperature differentiate in a more animal way than those reared at a temperature about 10°C higher (Hörstadius

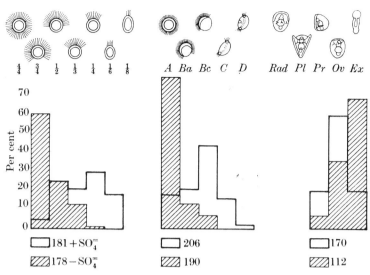

Fig. 82. Animalization of animal halves and vegetalization of vegetal halves of *Paracentrotus lividus* in SO₄-free sea-water. The columns indicate percentage, the numerals below the diagrams the number of halves in normal sea-water (heavy lines) and in SO₄-free sea-water (hatched). 4/4 and *Rad* are more-animal types than have ever been found among control halves. (Diagrams prepared after tables in Runnström *et al.* 1964.)

1949, Fig. 25). Recent investigations (Hörstadius 1973) have confirmed these results on animal halves and moreover have shown that the vegetal halves instead become clearly vegetalized at low temperature, thus proving the existence of two metabolically different systems. (This implies that the *an/veg* balance in the whole embryo probably remains unaltered at different temperatures.) It is hardly conceivable that one factor could have opposite effects at the poles of one gradient: the factor has evidently intervened in two different processes. The lack of sulphate has been interpreted as causing a lack of sulphated polysaccharides which in animal halves enhances, but in vegetal halves impairs, the interaction between cells (Immers and Runnström 1965, Runnström and Markman 1966).

In the search for inductive substances nucleic acids have attracted particular interest. The micromeres produce and contain a conspicuous amount of RNA (Agrell 1958; Cowden and Lehman 1963). Agrell (1956a) also found that the micromeres have a higher DNA-metabolism than the other blastomeres and ascribes the influence of the micromeres upon the polarity to an induction upon the mitotic state of the other cleavage cells. At the end of the 16-cell stage only the micromeres are synthesizing RNA, or at least they do so to a much greater extent than other blastomeres, and this RNA is necessary for the onset of gastrulation and differentiation of the archenteron (Czihak 1965a, b; Czihak, Wittman, and Hindennach 1967). Micromeres labelled with uridine-^{14}C were transplanted into unlabelled animal halves (Czihak and Hörstadius 1970). Labelled substance moved from the micromeres into the cytoplasm of the animal cells. Since the micromeres synthesize RNA it is probable that RNA is the substance that moves. It is tempting to combine this transport with the inductive action of the micromeres.

As to the transport and action of inductive substances, the following observation may be of interest. Animal cells treated with lithium can be incorporated in the blastula wall of animal halves and have the same capacity as micromeres to induce an archenteron and contribute to the

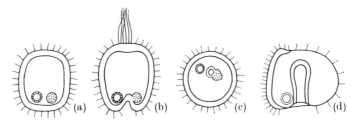

FIG. 83. An animal half into which two vegetal pieces from an animal half treated with lithium have been implanted. The invagination has started between the implants, none of them forming the tip of the archenteron. (From Hörstadius 1936b.)

formation of a pluteus (see Fig. 34). In one experiment two small pieces of the vegetal wall of a Li-treated animal half were implanted into an animal half. The one piece formed a small vesicle, the other a compact mass, both probably without a real fusion with the blastula wall (Fig. 83(a)). Then an invagination started between these two implants (b). The compact piece fused with a side of the archenteron (b), (c) and took part in the formation of its upper half. Even in the prism stage the vesicle was apparently lying free in the blastocoele (d). The question arose whether induction really occurred before fusion between implant and host. It was noteworthy that the invagination started between the implants, of which the one continuously appeared to lie free, and that the vegetalizing implant did not lead the invagination. The implant(s) evidently induced a region, the tip of the archenteron, which became more vegetal than the implant itself—an example of new polar concentration. This is different from implanted micromeres which represent the most vegetal material in the organism, themselves form primary mesenchyme cells, and, in some cases also, the archenteron tip.

There has been some discussion on the relation between cleavage and determination. The first four cleavages are synchronous. The formation of the four small micromeres occurs a little later than the other cell divisions (Theel 1892). According to Agrell (1956a, b, 1964) the synchronicity of mitotic events disappears during the following cleavages, a mitotic gradient spreading from the vegetal towards the animal pole, and the mitoses starting earlier in the vegetal half. The end of the synchronicity is combined with a change from utilizing cytoplasmic DNA to a new synthesis of nuclear DNA. Agrell considers that the induction of the mitotic state of the other blastomeres is brought about by the higher DNA-metabolism of the micromeres. He tentatively regards the graded mitotic activity as an actual cause of differentiation. He states, moreover, that the effect of lithium is a prolongation of the synchronous rhythm, without change of the mitotic rate but involving a prolonged utilization of the cytoplasmic DNA and the retardation of the new synthesis of nuclear DNA. A new mitotic gradient from the vegetal to the animal pole appears when the larva has reached the mesenchyme blastula stage (Agrell 1953); but this gradient, which is reverse to the mitochondrial gradient (see Fig. 35), develops too late to have bearing on the primary differentiation.

According to other, contrasting reports the rate of cleavage is retarded by lithium, while it is enhanced by the animalizing agents iodosobenzoic acid and trypsin (Hagström 1963; Hagström and Lönning 1963–5, 1967). These authors assume that the accelerated cleavage, which precedes animalization, promotes the increase in synthesis of DNA (and RNA) leading to an increased synthetic activity, and that consequently the slowly cleaving micromeres have a low synthesis. As external inducing substances are of disparate kinds and the only effect they seem to have in common is a change of cleavage rate, the same authors find it tempting to conclude that even minor changes in rate of cleavage will result in animalization or vegetalization. This idea is difficult to support. Protein synthesis is commonly assumed to take place during interphases rather than during mitoses. An increased number of cell divisions within a certain time span leads to shorter time of interphase periods and would consequently mean fewer syntheses.

Normal differentiation of whole eggs also occurs after an atypical sequence of cleavage divisions in relation to proceeding metabolic processes, as illustrated in Fig. 10. Plutei arise from eggs having passed through an equal cleavage, without formation of micro- and macromeres. Account must also be taken of all transplantations of halves, cell-rings, and micromeres, which have certainly upset the cleavage pattern in many ways and yet given results explicable in terms of gradients. In the many experiments with morphogenetically-active substances isolated from sea-urchin eggs (see page 168) it has been shown that some fractions cause animalization or vegetalization of animal and vegetal halves but not of whole embryos. On the other hand, animalization of whole embryos has been observed without corresponding effect on halves. Moreover, cases have been reported of agents causing animalization of animal halves and vegetalization of the vegetal halves by SO_4-free sea-water (Fig. 82, and by temperature, as reported above, p. 161) and, vice versa, vegetalization of animal halves in combination with animalization of the vegetal halves (Fig. 84(c)). These facts do not comply with the idea of cell divisions as governing differentiation: nearer to hand might be the concept of the mitotic activities and cell divisions as a result primarily of the metabolic processes in the cytoplasm. It is known that many substances interfere in very different, specific ways with the metabolism, and yet the result is often either animalization or vegetalization. It seems more probable that the cleavage divisions are guided by shift in either direction of the complex physiological processes, rather than the reverse. Indeed, in a review of cellular and molecular events associated with mitosis and meiosis, Stern (1970) when summing up certain investigations finds that the cytoplasm, during the nuclear phase of DNA synthesis, has the capacity to stimulate chromosomes to initiate replication, and as this capacity is not evident in the same cytoplasm at other phases of the cell cycle the conclusion is tentatively drawn that the onset of the S phase is due to some cytoplasmic transformation, the nature of which is not yet understood. In meiotic cells, at least, a number of specific syntheses occur in association with, and in anticipation of, chromosomal changes. In a chapter on nuclear-cytoplasmic transfers, Schjeide (1970) refers to cases where DNA synthesis appears to be regulated by cytoplasmic initiators.

In Chapter 5 it was reported that Boveri (1901*b*) explained the cleavage types by assuming that consecutive changes in the cytoplasm determine the position of the spindles. It was further stated that the vegetal cytoplasm is not activated to form micromeres until during the 8-cell stage (Hörstadius 1927, 1928). This conclusion was based on the formation of precocious micromeres in the 8-cell stage as a result of delayed cleavage (see Fig. 10), and particularly on the fact that micromeres do not appear in the 8-cell stage of ventral halves isolated before fertilization although the spindles in their 4-cell stage occupy about the same position as in the vegetal blastomeres of a normal 8-cell stage (cf. Fig 11(e)$_4$ and 10(a)$_5$). Rustad (1960) delayed cleavages by X-ray irradiation without affecting the micromere clock (Dan and Ikeda 1971). They advance the hypothesis that the clock system is related to rhythmical fluctuations of the sulfhydryl content of the egg proteins. Ultraviolet radiation interrupts cleavage without affecting the SH-rhythm. When exactly one early cell cycle was skipped precocious micromeres appeared as expected. When reagents (NaN$_3$, puromycin) were used stopping both SH-changes and cleavage simultaneously, no micromeres were pinched off in the 8-cell stage after release of the standstill. In a third series the SH-cycle was stopped by ethyl ether. This reagent does not interfere with the nuclear divisions. At the cleavage to 16 cells the SH-clock had not yet struck for micromere formation. The results thus came out as anticipated by the hypothesis. The idea that changes in time between SH-cycle and cell divisions should have a bearing on the segregation of animal and vegetal materials (Dan 1972) is hardly acceptable. As emphasized in the above paragraph typical development proceeds independently of the type of cleavage.

The process of regeneration has been studied particularly in amphibians. One theory of the sources of regenerative material has been that the tissues in the regenerated part arise from corresponding tissues in the remainder of the organ. However, observations have shown that the new tissues are derived from cells which undergo a true differentiation. Cells have been thought to remain in an embryonic stage as a reserve. In modern terms (Scarano 1969), the diverse capacities for regeneration might depend on an early cessation of sequential steps of DNA modifications during organogenesis. Modern investigations, however, indicate radical breakdown of tissues in the wound and suggest the possibility that, in this connexion, cells become de-differentiated yet retain embryonic faculties of differentiation into several types of tissue cells. Regeneration would thus imply a de-differentiation followed by a re-differentiation. In the light of these opinions it may be worth while to recall the observations illustrated in Figs. 58, 59, 65(d), 66(b), 67(f) and (g). These do not accord with any of the above theories. Coelom can be regenerated from already-differentiated embryonic germ layers, bulging out from the ectoderm, oesophagus and stomach, or formed by the association of mesenchyme cells. When coelom originates in the ectoderm or endoderm epithelia no breakdown of cells nor use of other cells has been observed: the regeneration seems to occur by a direct re-differentiation.

Analysis of the physiological basis of determination and differentiation encounters enormous difficulties in interpretation of the results. A shift in the *an/veg* balance may depend on enhancement of the vegetal or impairment of the animal system, or vice versa. This is evidenced by the following experiments. When implanted micromeres induce an archenteron in animal halves we are evidently dealing with suppression of animal properties as a consequence of increased vegetal forces. However, when implantation of micromeres in the animal pole of an animal half results in gastrulation also at the vegetal side (see Fig. 21(c), $(g)_3$) the authentic reinforcement of the vegetal gradient is due to weakening of the animal properties. Lallier (1955) has shown that zinc ions act strongly in an animalizing manner. From further experiments (1959a) he states, plausibly enough, that the zinc ions do not directly strengthen the animal gradient, but instead they primarily attack the vegetal region and thereby allow the animal system to predominate.

The reason for the widespread use of animal and vegetal halves for testing the effect of substances is that the gradient system is rather stable in whole eggs and that small changes—for example, the volume of material in the digestive tract—are difficult to discern. In whole larvae, an intensification of either animal or vegetal properties is often first perceivable as a radialization. In halves, on the other hand, the balance is very labile and small deviations give rise to a number of clearly distinguishable types (see Fig. 13).

The very extensive literature on the physiology of normal echinoid development—for example, the gradual changes in metabolism without direct bearing on determination—falls outside the scope of this study. An attempt to cover physiological, biochemical, and molecular works which try to throw light on determination and differentiation would also lengthen the book intolerably without giving an acceptable picture of this very complex field. However, as this book is devoted to experiments chiefly made with mechanical means, and as fragments have proved valuable because of their sensitivity, it may be permissible to give a list of references to those investigations in which isolations have rendered service as tools. The list is presented without discussion of the interpretations of the results. For reviews of echinoid developmental physiology or parts thereof see, for example, Czihak 1971, Gustafson 1965, 1969, Lallier 1964, Ranzi 1962, Runnström 1966b, Tyler and

Tyler 1966; and for cell differentiation in general, Ebert and Sussex 1970, Schjeide and De Vellis 1970.

von Ubisch (1925*c*, *d*, 1929) showed that the classical vegetalizing agent LiCl can transform animal halves to gastrulae, plutei, and exogastrulae. Compared to animalizing substances the vegetalizing ones are rather few. Phenazone and chloramphenicol are vegetalizers (Lallier 1959*b*, 1962), the latter, which is an inhibitor of protein metabolism, also has a strong effect on animal halves (Hörstadius 1963). Dinitrophenol, known as an inhibitor of oxydative phosphorylation, also has the power of making plutei of animal halves but the effect is very varied, some of the halves often remaining as blastulae (Hörstadius 1953*c*). Fourteen amino acids were found to bring about a slight vegetal trend while glutamine and lysine gave a clear animalization (Hörstadius and Strömberg 1940; Hörstadius and Gustafson 1948; Hörstadius 1949; Gustafson and Hörstadius 1957). D- and L-*p*-tyrosine, *o*-tyrosine, and *m*-tyrosine have later been found to have a vegetalizing effect on whole embryos also (Mastrangelo 1966). Several antimetabolites had similar effects, namely analogues to vitamin B6, cysteine, niacin, phenylalanine, while analogues to ascorbic acid, adenine, guanine, uracil, cytosine (strong effect also on whole eggs), and niacin were animalizing (thus antimetabolites to niacin could act in both directions; compare the double effect of lack of sulphate and of CO, mentioned earlier in this chapter) (Hörstadius and Gustafson 1954; Gustafson and Hörstadius 1955, 1956). Chloroxanthine, an antimetabolite to purines and nucleic acid, animalized whole eggs also, even after treatment before fertilization (Hörstadius and Gustafson 1954). Animal halves became more or less animalized when reared in solutions of DNA isolated from sea-urchin sperm, and also in three of five tested synthetic nucleosides (Hörstadius, Lorch, and Chargaff 1954). Lindberg (1943, 1945, 1946) found that the degradation of carbohydrate through phosphorylated substances in the sea-urchin embryos takes, on the whole, another course than in muscle, and he synthesized the new phosphate ester involved, 1,2-propanediol phosphate. Both this ester and also phosphogluconic acid, lactate, and sodium pyruvate were shown to act as animalizers (Hörstadius and Gustafson 1947; Hörstadius and Strömberg 1940). The proteolytic enzymes trypsin and ficin were found to be strong animalizers (Hörstadius 1953*c*, 1965*a*), the former transforming vegetal halves not only into plutei but also into larvae of more animal type. Pronase, papaine, and chymopapaine animalize whole eggs (Lallier 1969).

In order to study regional differences in early development, incorporations of labelled nucleic acids, proteins, amino acids, and SO_4 were made into halves (Markman 1962, 1967; Runnström *et al.* 1964; Berg 1965, 1968; Hörstadius *et al.* 1966). The effect of actinomycin on halves was reported by Markman (1963), Markman and Runnström (1963, 1970), de Angelis and Runnström (1970), and on the potentialities of animal halves in combination with micromeres by Giudice and Hörstadius (1965).

No marked difference in the rate of protein synthesis nor in cytochrome oxidase activities was found among large quantities of chemically-isolated micromeres, macromeres, and mesomeres (Spiegel and Tyler 1966; Berg 1958). An extraordinary phenomenon is demonstrated by still smaller isolated cells, dissociated as late as in blastula or pluteus stages. Large quantities brought closely together in normal sea-water started quickly to reaggregate and form structures which differentiated into quasi-normal larvae (Giudice 1962). Cells isolated from blastulae vegetalized by LiCl reaggregated into lumps of cells of vegetal character but without forming archenteron or skeleton. They almost completely lacked an external epithelial lining. Those animalized by $ZnSO_4$ gave rise to ciliated spheres. The reaggregated cells have, therefore, retained their induced vegetal and animal character (Giudice 1963).

No difference in respiration was found between animal and vegetal halves isolated at 16-cell stages and measured in the microrespirometer of Linderström–Lang at from 6 to 28 hours after fertilization (Lindahl and Holter 1940). The release of maximal respiration by dinitrophenol was studied in halves and gave different results in early stages and in mesenchyme blastulae (De Vincentiis *et al.* 1966). The many investigations on respiration in sea-urchin larvae have given rather bewildering, sometimes contradictory, results: in this chapter it is not possible to enter further upon this field.

Since implantation of vegetal cytoplasm as well as the rearing of embryos in mixtures of segregated micromeres produced no effect (see page 72), and since application of external agents means rather artificial encroachments, a new approach was attempted by searching for morphogenetically-active substances in the sea-urchin eggs themselves. A great many fractions were separated on Dowex and on Sephadex, and were tested on halves and whole larvae; some of these endogenous substances appeared to be morphogenetically active (Hörstadius *et al.* 1967; Josefsson and Hörstadius 1969; Hörstadius and Josefsson 1972). The diagrams (see Fig. 84) show how the percentage of larval types in the presence of two fractions has moved in (respectively) animal (a) and

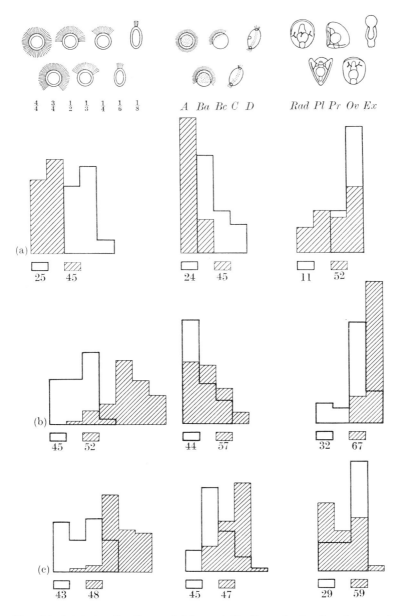

FIG. 84. (a) Animalization and (b) vegetalization of animal and vegetal halves by two substances isolated from eggs of the same species, *Paracentrotus lividus*. (c) Vegetalization of the animal halves and animalization of the vegetal halves by a third substance. Control halves: heavy lines. Treated halves: hatched. ((a) from Josefsson and Hörstadius 1969; (b), (c) unpublished.)

vegetal (b) direction as compared to the controls. Fig. 84(c) illustrates vegetalization of animal and animalization of vegetal halves by a third fraction, a result the reverse of, for example, the effect of SO_4-free sea-water (see Fig. 82). Larvae were discovered which were more animal than any among the controls (animal tuft 4/4; vegetal halves with enlarged tuft and with radial symmetry, *Rad*). In one experiment the anal arms of vegetal halves reached an abnormal length, resulting in a

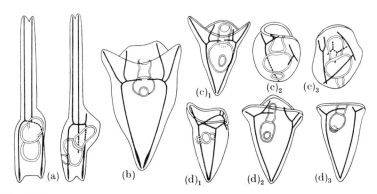

FIG. 85. (a) Two vegetal halves with extraordinarily long anal arms after treatment with an endogenous fraction. (b)–(d) Experiments with endo-genous substances causing reduction of the endoderm without expected corresponding strong animalizing effect on bilateral symmetry of ecto-derm and skeleton. (b) Whole larva. (c) Control vegetal halves. (d) Vegetal halves with much reduced endoderm. ((a) from Hörstadius and Josefsson 1972, (b)–(d) from Hörstadius 1972.)

larval shape never observed before (Fig. 85(a)), and in other cases a strong reduction of the endoderm in whole eggs and in vegetal halves was not accompanied by the expected corresponding effect on the ecto-derm and skeleton (b)–(d). Some of the fractions caused whole eggs to form larvae with enlarged tuft and diminished archenteron, as well as exogastrulae with large archenteron. See also Fig. 25. The effect of animalizing and vegetalizing substances was neutralized when these were applied simultaneously. The character of the active substances has not yet been analysed, but the ultra-violet absorption curves of two animalizing agents resemble those of tryptophane and of adenine.

The animalizing effect of one of the endogenous morphogenetic fractions, as well as of trypsin, was removed, or almost removed, by actinomycin D (Fig. 86) (Markman and Runnström 1970). Similarly, actinomycin D counteracted the vegetalization of animal halves by lithium (de Angelis and Runnström 1970). From these experiments the authors infer that the agents in question control the transcription of genes specifying the differentiation in the animal or vegetal direction.

Excessive condensation in summaries may mislead the reader concerning the point involved. The presentation of the conclusion in the last two papers mentioned may be interpreted as speaking for a direct effect of the agents on the gene molecules. However, it is not plausible that several substances of quite different nature could activate the same genes, and

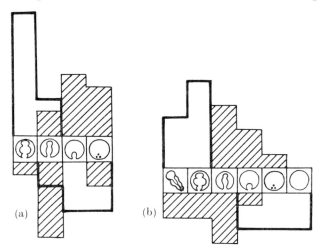

FIG. 86. (a) Histogram showing as abscissa four different types of differentiation of vegetal halves and, as ordinate, the frequency of these types under different experimental conditions. Upward-directed columns refer to control halves (heavy lines) or to halves reared in sea-water + actinomycin D (hatched). Downward-directed columns refer to embryos reared in a solution of an endogenous animalizing fraction (heavy outline), or to animalizing fraction + actinomycin D (hatched). (b) Trypsin used as animalizing agent. (From Markman and Runnström 1970.)

do so in the form of gradients. We know (as elaborated on page 137) that the early development depends on the location of the nuclei within the egg regions, where they will be surrounded by a cytoplasm of special structure and metabolism—in sea-urchins, with a certain *an/veg* balance. Foreign agents interfere in different ways in the complex physiology of the cell, some of them, nevertheless, with the same result, enhancing or impairing animal and vegetal processes and thereby evoking different parts of the genome. This basic idea is, indeed, clearly elaborated in papers by Runnström on the mechanism of control of differentiation (1964, 1966*b*, 1967; also Czihak 1968 and, more biochemically, Scarano 1971). For reviews of cytoplasmic control of nuclear activities, see Gurdon and Woodland (1968) and Denis (1970).

Another example of cytoplasmic influences is provided by transplantations of sea-urchin blastomeres. Animal cells have cytoplasm and nuclei destined to form ectoderm, but implanted micromeres convert them into endoderm as a result of information, the first step in a determination process, which must have reached the presumptive ectoderm nuclei via the cytoplasm. A stream of substance which might fulfil the requirements of such moving information or induction has been visualized by implanting micromeres labelled with uridine into unlabelled animal halves, as mentioned earlier in this chapter.

In our era of genes and nucleic acids the preceding two paragraphs may be presented as a tribute to the cytoplasm. This paragraph, on the other hand, will take up the cudgels for the nucleus and discuss the remarkable capacity of embryos at cleavage stages to get rid of undesirable foreign bodies by ejecting them (see Fig. 30) or by making them fall out through an opening between the blastomeres. The process consists of three steps: (a) the ability of the embryo to perceive the difference on the one hand, between micromeres of its own or closely-related species and micromeres of a sea-urchin of another order (see page 155) and, on the other hand, between micromeres of its own species and vegetal cytoplasm without nuclei (see page 72); (b) while implanted micromeres of its own or closely related species within a very short time fuse with the host cells after disintegration of parts of the cell membranes, the undesirable implants remain unattached—otherwise they could not be rejected; (c) the double modes of rejection.

What process enables the blastomeres to sense as unwelcome intruders the order-alien micromeres, but not those from more closely-related species? This might be a matter of immunological rejection. In the experiments illustrated in Fig. 30, the implanted cytoplasm had been isolated shortly before from a fertilized egg of the same species. This cytoplasm is no dead body. It is known that enucleated eggs can be fertilized and can develop (merogones) and that they can also be parthenogenetically activated and can divide (see pp. 81, 141). Furthermore, in contrast to cytolysing eggs they are not permeable to trypan blue (see page 73). Is it possible to imagine an immunological reaction between cells and cytoplasm of the same species when no such reaction occurs between intact cells? If not, which kind of reaction is at work here? In any case, the experiments show that as early as the first hours of life in a zygote the activity of the nucleus is imperative for the maintenance of normal properties in the cytoplasm.

One last question. When a vegetal half was transplanted on top of another vegetal half (see Fig. 26) a reorganization within the animal–vegetal system did not occur in the line of the two joint axes, as might have been expected in view of other experiments (see for example, Fig. 21 and Fig. 28(c)). Instead, the upper half moved down along the lower partner until the endodermal regions fused. What kind of reaction and what forces caused this strange migration ?

References

AGRELL, E. (1953). *Ark. Zool.* **6**, 213.

—— (1956a). *Bertil Hanström. Zool. papers* (ed. *Wingstrand*). Lund. p. 27.

—— (1956b). *Acta zool., Stockh.* **37**, 33.

—— (1958). *Ark. Zool.* **11**, 435.

—— (1964). *Synchrony in cell division and growth* (ed. *E. Zeuthen*). p. 39. John Wiley and Sons, New York.

ALLEN, R. D. and HAGSTRÖM, B. (1955). *Exptl Cell Res., Suppl.* **3**, 1.

BÄCKSTRÖM, S. (1961). *Reducing agents and activities in sea urchin development.* Uppsala.

—— (1963). *Acta Embryol. Morph. exp.* **6**, 235.

BÄCKSTRÖM, S., HULTIN, S., and HULTIN, T. (1960). *Exptl Cell Res.* **19**, 634.

BALINSKY, S. (1932). *Zh. bio. -zool. Tsyklu, Kyev.* no. **1–2**, 5.

BALTZER, F. (1910). *Arch. Zellforsch.* **5**, 497.

—— (1920). *Verh. schweiz. naturf. Ges.* **101**, 217.

—— (1930). *Revue suisse Zool.* **37**, 525.

—— (1940). *Naturwissenschaften.* **28**, 196.

BALTZER, F. and CHEN, P. S. (1960). *Revue suisse Zool.* **67**, 183.

—— —— (1965). *Experientia.* **21**, 194.

BALTZER, F., CHEN, P. S. and TARDENT, P. (1961). *Jber. schweiz. Ges. Vererbungs.* **36**, 126.

BALTZER, F., TARDENT, P. and CHEN, P. S. (1967). *Experientia.* **23**, 777.

BARROIS, S. (1888). *Rec. Zool. Suisse.* **4**, 545.

BARROS, C. G. S., HAND, JR., and MONROY, A. (1966). *Exptl Cell Res.* **43**, 167.

BATAILLON, E. (1900). *C. r. hebd. Séanc. Acad. Sci., Paris.* **130**, 1201.

BERG, W. E. (1958). *Exptl Cell Res.* **50**, 679.

—— (1965). *Exptl Cell Res.* **40**, 469.

—— (1968). *Exptl Cell Res.* **50**, 679.

BERG, W. E. and CHENG, A. G. (1962). *Acta Embryol. Morph. exp.* **5**, 167.

BERG, W. E., TAYLOR, D. A., and HUMPHREYS, W. J. (1962). *Devl Biol.* 4, 165.

BIERENS DE HAAN, J. A. (1913a). *Arch. EntwMech. Org.* **36**, 473.

—— (1913b). *Arch. EntwMech. Org.* **37**, 420.

—— (1913c). *Zool. Anz.* **42**, 500.

BORCEA, M. I. (1909). *C. r. hebd. Séanc. Acad. Sci., Paris.* **149**, 637.

BOVERI, T. (1887). *Anat. Anz.* **2**, 688.

—— (1889). *S. B. Ges. Morph. Physiol. München.* **5**, 73.

—— (1890). *Jena Z. Naturw.* **24**, 314.

—— (1895). *Arch. EntwMech. Org.* **2**, 394.

—— (1901a). *Zool. Jb. Abt. Anat. Ont.* **14**, 630.

—— (1901b). *Verh. phys. med. Ges. Würzb.* **34**, 145.

—— (1902). *Verh. phys. med. Ges. Würzb.* **35**, 67.

BOVERI, T. (1903). *S. B. phys. med. Ges. Würzb., Jahrg.* **1903**, 12.

—— (1904*a*). *S. B. phys. med. Ges. Würzb. Jahrbg.* 1904.

—— (1904*b*) *Ergebnisse über die Konstitution der chromatischen Substanz des Zellkerns.* Gustav Fischer, Jena.

—— (1905). *Jena Z. Naturw.* **39**, 445.

—— (1908). *Jena Z. Naturw.* **43**, 1.

—— (1910*a*). *Festschrift für Richard Hertwig.* **3**, 131.

—— (1910*b*). *Arch. EntwMech. Org.* **30**, 2, 101.

—— (1914*a*). *Verh. phys. med. Ges. Würzb.* **43**, 117.

—— (1914*b*). *Zur Frage der Entstehung maligner Tumoren.* Gustav Fischer, Jena.

—— (1918). *Arch. EntwMech. Org.* **44**, 417.

BRACHET, J. (1970). *Ann. Biol.* **9**, 619.

—— (1971*a*). *Proc. R. Soc., Lond.* **B 178**, 227.

—— (1971*b*). In *Cours et document de biologie*, Vol. 2. Gordon and Breach, Paris, p. 330.

—— DECROLY, M., FICQ, A., and QUERTIER, J. (1963). *Biochim. biophys. Acta* **72**, 660.

BRIGGS, R. *and* KING, T. J. (1952). *Proc. natn. Acad. Sci. U.S.A.* **38**, 455.

BURY, H. (1888). *Phil. Trans. R. Soc.* **B. 179**, 257.

BÜTSCHLI, O. (1915). *S. B. Akad. Wiss. Heidelberg.* **6B**, 1.

CALLAN, H. G. (1914). *Biochim. biophys. Acta* **3**, 92.

CARPENTER, W. (1866). *Phil. Trans. R. Soc.* **156**, 671.

CAVANAUGH, G. M. (1956). *Formulae and methods of the marine biol. lab. chemical room. Woods Hole, Mass. U.S.A.*

CHABRY, L. (1887). *J. Anat. Physiol. Lond.* **23**, 167.

CHAMBERS, R. (1921). *Biol. Bull. mar. biol. Lab., Woods Hole.* **41**, 318.

CHEN, P. S. *and* BALTZER, F. (1962). *Experientia.* **18**, 522.

—— —— (1964). *Experientia.* **20**, 236.

CHILD, C. M. (1907). *Arch. EntwMech. Org.* **24**, 315.

—— (1915). *Am. J. Physiol.* **37**, 203.

—— (1916*a*). *J. Morph.* **28**, 65.

—— (1916*b*). *Biol. Bull. mar. biol. Lab., Woods Hole*, **30**, 391.

—— (1936). *W. Roux. Arch. EntwMech. Org.* **135**, 426.

—— (1941). *Patterns and problems of development.* University of Chicago Press.

CHUN, C. (1892). *Festschrift für R. Leuckart.* Leipzig, p. 77.

CONKLIN, E. G. (1905*a*). *Biol. Bull. mar. biol. Lab., Woods Hole.* **8**, 205.

—— (1905*b*). *J. Acad. nat. Sci. Philad.* **13**, 1.

—— (1906). *Arch. EntwMech. Org.* **21**, 727.

COWDEN, R. R. *and* LEHMAN, H. E. (1963). *Growth.* **27**, 185.

CZIHAK, G. (1961). *W. Roux Arch. EntwMech. Org.* **153**, 353.

—— (1962). *W. Roux Arch. EntwMech. Org.* **154**, 29.

—— (1963). *W. Roux Arch. EntwMech. Org.* **154**, 272.

—— (1965*a*). *W. Roux Arch. EntwMech. Org.* **155**, 709.

—— (1965*b*). *W. Roux Arch. EntwMech. Org.* **156**, 504.

—— (1966). *W. Roux Arch. EntwMech. Org.* **157**, 199.

—— (1968). *Pubbl. Staz. zool. Napoli.* **36**, 321.

—— (1971). Echinoids. In *Experimental embryology of marine and fresh water invertebrates* (ed. G. Reverberi). North Holland Pub. Co., Amsterdam, p. 363.

CZIHAK, G. *and* HÖRSTADIUS, S. (1970). Devl Biol. **22**, 15.

CZIHAK, G., WITTMAN, H. G. *and* HINDENNACH, I. (1967). *Z. Naturf.* **22b**, 1176.

DALCQ, A. (1941). *L'oeuf et son dynamisme organisateur.* Paris.

DAN, J. C. (1956). *Int. Rev. Cytol.* **5**, 365.

DAN, K. (1960). *Int. Rev. Cytol.* **9**, 321.

—— (1972). *Exptl Cell Res.* **72**, 69.

—— and IKEDA, M. (1971). *Develop. Growth and Different.* **13**, 285.

DAN, K. and OKAZAKI, K. (1956). *Biol. Bull. mar. biol. Lab., Woods Hole.* **110**, 29.

DE ANGELIS, E. and RUNNSTRÖM, J. (1970). *W. Roux Arch. EntwMech. Org.* **164**, 236.

DELAGE, Y. (1899). *Archs. Zool. exp. gén., ser.* 3, **7**, 383.

DENIS, H. (1970). *Archs int. Physiol. Biochim.* **78**, 367.

DENIS, H. and BRACHET, J. (1969a). *Proc. natn. Acad. Sci., U.S.A.* **62**, 194.

—— —— (1969b). *Proc. natn. Acad. Sci., U.S.A.* **62**, 438.

—— —— (1970). *Eur. J. Biochem.* **13**, 86.

DERBÈS, M. (1847). *Annls Sci. nat., Zool.* **8**, 80.

DE VINCENTIIS, S., HÖRSTADIUS, S. and RUNNSTRÖM, J. (1966). *Exptl. cell Res.* **41**, 535.

DRIESCH, H. (1891). *Z. wiss. Zool.* **53**, 160.

—— (1892). *Z. wiss. Zool.* **55**, 1.

—— (1893a). *Mitt. Zool. Stat. Neapel.* **11**, 221.

—— (1893b). *Anat. Anz.* **8**, 348.

—— (1893c). *Biol. Zbl.* **13**, 296.

—— (1895). *Arch. EntwMech. Org.* **2**, 169.

—— (1896a). *Arch. EntwMech. Org.* **3**, 362.

—— (1896b). *Arch. EntwMech. Org.* **4**, 75.

—— (1896c). *Arch. EntwMech. Org.* **4**, 247.

—— (1898a). *Arch. EntwMech. Org.* **6**, 198.

—— (1898b). *Arch. EntwMech. Org.* **7**, 65.

—— (1899a). *Arch. EntwMech. Org.* **8**, 35.

—— (1899b). *Arch. EntwMech. Org.* **9**, 137.

—— (1900a). *Arch. EntwMech. Org.* **10**, 361.

—— (1900b). *Arch. EntwMech. Org.* **10**, 411.

—— (1901). *Die organischen Regulationen.* Leipzig.

—— (1902). *Arch. EntwMech. Org.* **14**, 500.

—— (1903). *Arch. EntwMech. Org.* **17**, 41.

—— (1904). *Arch. EntwMech. Org.* **17**, 306.

—— (1905). *Arch. EntwMech. Org.* **19**, 658.

—— (1906). *Arch. EntwMech. Org.* **21**, 756.

—— (1908). *Arch. EntwMech. Org.* **26**, 130.

—— (1910). *Arch. EntwMech. Org.* **30**, 8.

DRIESCH, H. and MORGAN, T. H. (1895). *Arch. EntwMech. Org.* **2**, 204.

EBERT, J. D. and SUSSEX, I. M. (1970). *Interacting systems in development.* Holt, Rinehart, and Winston, New York.

ENDO, Y. (1952). *Exptl Cell Res.* **3**, 406.

—— (1961a). *Exptl Cell Res.* **25**, 383.

—— (1961b). *Exptl Cell Res.* **25**, 518.

FICQ, A. and BRACHET, J. (1963). *Exptl Cell Res.* **32**, 90.

FIEDLER, K. (1891). *Festschr. f. Nägeli u. Kölliker.* Zürich, p. 191.

FISCHEL, A. (1909). *Arch. EntwMech. Org.* **27**, 465.

FOERSTER, M. and ÖRSTRÖM, Å. (1933). *Trav. Stn. biol. Roscoff,* **11**, 63.

FOL, H. (1877). *Archs zool. exp. gén.* **6**, 145.

—— (1879). *Mém. Soc. Phys. Hist. nat. Genève,* **26**, 89.

FRY, H. (1924). *Anat. Rec.* **28**, 371.

—— (1927) *Biol. Bull. mar. biol. Lab., Woods Hole,* **53**, 173.

GARBOWSKI, M. T. (1904). *Bull. intn. Acad. Sci. Cracovie,* 169.

GARBOWSKI, M. T. (1905) *Bull. int. Acad. Sci. Cracovie*, 599.

GINSBURG, A. S. (1968). *Fertilization in fishes and the problem of polyspermy.* Publishing House Nauka. Moskwa.

GIUDICE, G. (1962). *Devl Biol.* **5**, 402.

—— (1963). *Experientia.* **19**, 83.

GIUDICE, G. and HÖRSTADIUS, S. (1965). *Exptl Cell Res.* **39**, 117.

GIUDICE, G., MUTOLO, V. and DONATUTI, G. (1968). *W. Roux Arch. Entw Mech. Org.* **41**, 579.

GLISIN, V. R. and GLISIN, M. V. (1964). *Proc. natn. Acad. Sci. U.S.A.* **52**, 1523.

—— —— (1964). *Proc. natn. Acad. Sci., U.S.A.* **52**, 1548.

GOLDFORB, A. J. (1914). *Arch. EntwMech. Org.* **41**, 579.

—— (1917) *Biol. Bull. mar. biol. Lab. Woods Hole*, **32**, 21.

GURDON, J. B. (1968). *Scient. Am.* **219**, 24.

GURDON, J. B. and WOODLAND, H. R. (1968). *Biol. Rev.* **43**, 233.

GUSTAFSON, T. (1945). *Ark. Zool.* **B37**, 1.

—— (1946). *Ark. Zool.* **A38**, no. 4.

—— (1952). *Ark. Zool., Ser.* 2, **3**, 273.

—— (1963). *Exptl Cell Res.* **32**, 570.

—— (1965). In *The biochemistry of animal development* (*ed. R. Wever*). Vol. 1, part 2, 140.

—— (1969). In *Chemical Zoology*, Vol. 3. Academic Press, New York, p. 149.

GUSTAFSON, T. and HÖRSTADIUS, S. (1955). *Exptl Cell Res. Suppl.* **3**, 170.

—— —— (1956). *Zool. Anz.* **156**, 102.

—— —— (1957). *Pubbl. Staz. zool. Napoli*, **29**, 407.

GUSTAFSON, T. and KINNANDER, H. (1960). *Exptl Cell Res.* **21**, 361.

GUSTAFSON, T. and LENIQUE, P. (1952). *Exptl Cell Res.* **3**, 251.

GUSTAFSON, T. and SÄVHAGEN, R. (1949). *Ark. Zool.* **A42**, no. 10.

GUSTAFSON, T. and TONEBY, M. (1971). *Am. Scient.* **59**, 452.

GUSTAFSON, T. and WOLPERT, L. (1961). *Exptl Cell Res.* **22**, 509.

—— —— (1963). *Int. Rev. Cytol.* **15**, 139.

—— —— (1967). *Biol. Rev.* **42**, 442.

HADORN, E. (1930). *Rev. suisse Zool.* **37**, 333.

—— (1932). *W. Roux Arch. EntwMech. Org.* **125**, 495.

—— (1936). *Verh. dt. Zool. Ges.*, 97.

—— (1937). *W. Roux Arch. EntwMech. Org.* **136**, 400.

HAGSTRÖM, B. E. (1956*a*). *Exptl Cell Res.* **10**, 24.

—— (1956*b*). *Exptl Cell Res.* **10**, 740.

—— (1956*c*). *The role of the jelly coat and the block to polyspermy in the fertilization of sea urchins.* Almqvist a. Wiksell. Uppsala.

—— (1959). *Exptl Cell Res.* **17**, 256.

—— (1963). *Biol. Bull. mar. biol. Lab., Woods Hole*, **124**, 55.

HAGSTRÖM, B. E. and LÖNNING, S. (1963). *Ark. Zool.* **15**, 377.

—— —— (1964). *Sarsia.* **15**, 17.

—— —— (1965). *Sarsia.* **18**, 1.

—— —— (1967). *W. Roux Arch. EntwMech. Org.* **158**, 1.

—— —— (1969). *Protoplasma*, **68**, 271.

HARRIS, H. (1971). *Proc. R. Soc., Lond.* **B 179**, 1.

HARVEY, E. B. (1933). *Biol. Bull. mar. biol. Lab., Woods Hole*, **64**, 125.

—— (1936). *Biol. Bull. mar. biol. Lab., Woods Hole*, **71**, 101.

—— (1956). *The American Arbacia and other sea urchins.* Princeton Univ. Press.

HARVEY, E. N. (1910). *J. exp. Zool.* **8**, 355.

HEFFNER, B. (1908). *Arch. EntwMech. Org.* **26**, 1.

HERBST, C. (1892). *Z. wiss. Zool.* **55**, 446.
—— (1893). *Mitt. zool. Stn. Neapel.* **11**, 136.
—— (1895). *Biol. Zbl.* **15**, 720.
—— (1896). *Arch. EntwMech. Org.* **2**, 455.
—— (1897). *Arch. EntwMech. Org.* **5**, 649.
—— (1900). *Arch. EntwMech. Org.* **9**, 424.
—— (1904). *Arch. EntwMech. Org.* **17**, 306.
—— (1906a). *Arch. EntwMech. Org.* **21**, 173.
—— (1906b). *Arch. EntwMech. Org.* **22**, 473.
—— (1907). *Arch. EntwMech. Org.* **24**, 185.
—— (1909). *Arch. EntwMech. Org.* **27**, 266.
—— (1912). *Arch. EntwMech. Org.* **34**, 1.
—— (1913). *Sber. heidelb. Akad. Wiss.* **B**, Jg. 1913, 81.
—— (1914). *Arch. EntwMech. Org.* **39.**, 617.
—— (1926). *Handb. norm. patholog. Physiol.* **17**, Frankfurt am Main.
HERTWIG, O. (1876). *Gegenbaurs morphol. Jb.* **1**, 347.
—— (1885). *Jena Z. Naturwiss.* **18**, 175.
—— (1890). *Arch. mikrosk. Anat.* **36**, 1.
HERTWIG, O. and HERTWIG, R. (1887). *Jena Z. Naturwiss.* **20**, 120.
HERTWIG, R. (1903). *Biol. Zbl.* **23**, 49.
HINDERER, T. (1914). *Arch. EntwMech. Org.* **38**, 187 and 364.
HINEGARDNER, R. (1973). In press, in *The sea urchin embryo. Biochemistry and morphogenesis* (Ed. *G. Czihak*). Springer Verlag.
HIRAMOTO, Y. (1954). *Jap. J. Zool.* **11**, 227.
—— (1955a). *Jap. J. Zool.* **11**, 333.
—— (1955b) *Annotnes zool. jap.* **28**, 183.
—— (1962). *Exptl Cell Res.* **27**, 416.
HIS, W. (1874). *Unsere Körperform und das physiologische Problem ihrer Entstehung.* Verlag Vogel, Leipzig.
HÖRSTADIUS, S. (1925a). *Ark. Zool.* **B17**, no. 6.
—— (1925b). *Ark. Zool.* **B17**, no. 7.
—— (1925c). *Ark. Zool.* **B17**, no. 8.
—— (1925d). *Biologia gen.* **1**, 522.
—— (1927). *W. Roux Arch. EntwMech. Org.* **112**, 239.
—— (1928). *Acta zool., Stockh.* **9**, 1.
—— (1931). *Ark. Zool.* **B23**, no. 1.
—— (1932). *Naturwissenschaften.* **20**, 363.
—— (1935). *Pubbl. Stn. zool., Napoli,* **14**, 251.
—— (1936a). *W. Roux Arch. EntwMech. Org.* **135**, 1.
—— (1936b). *W. Roux Arch. EntwMech. Org.* **135**, 40.
—— (1936c). *Mém. Mus. r. Hist. nat. Belg. Ser.* 2, **3**, 801.
—— (1937). *Biol. Bull. mar. biol. Lab., Woods Hole,* **73**, 295.
—— (1938). *W. Roux Arch. EntwMech. Org.* **138**, 197.
—— (1939a). *Biol. Rev.* **14**, 132.
—— (1939b). *Pubbl. Stn. zool., Napoli,* **17**, 221.
—— (1949). *Pubbl. Stn. zool., Napoli, Suppl.* **21**, 131.
—— (1950a). *J. exp. Zool.* **113**, 245.
—— (1950b). *Année biol.* **26**, 381.
—— (1950c). *The neural crest. Its properties and derivatives in the light of experimental research.* Oxford University Press, London.
—— (1952). *J. exp. Zool.* **120**, 421.
—— (1953a). *Pubbl. Stn. zool., Napoli,* **24**, 45.

HÖRSTADIUS, S. (1953*b*). *J. Embryol. exp. Morph.* **1**, 257.
—— (1953*c*). *J. Embryol. exp. Morph.* **1**, 327.
—— (1955). *J. exp. Zool.* **129**, 249.
—— (1957). *J. Embryol. exp. Morph.* **5**, 60.
—— (1959). *J. exp. Zool.* **142**, 141.
—— (1960). *Symp. Germ Cells.* Fondazione Baselli, Milano, p. 384.
—— (1961). *Embryologia.* **6**, 119.
—— (1962). *Symp. genet. Biol. Italica,* **9**, 1.
—— (1963). *Devl Biol.* **7**, 144.
—— (1965*a*). *Zool. Jb. Physiol.* **71**, 241.
—— (1965*b*). *Z. Naturf.* **20B**, 331.
—— (1966). *Arch. zool. Ital.* **51**, 433.
—— (1971). *Ark. Zool. Ser.* 2, **23**, 417.
—— (1972). *Exptl Cell Res.* **72**, 140.
—— (1973). In press in *Exptl Cell Res.* **78**.
HÖRSTADIUS, S. *and* GUSTAFSON, T. (1947). *Zool. Bidr., Uppsala.* **25**, 571.
—— —— (1948). *Symp. Soc. exp. Biol.* **2**, Growth in relation to differentiation and morphogenesis. Cambridge, p. 50.
—— —— (1954). *J. Embryol. exp. Morph.* **2**, 216.
HÖRSTADIUS, S., IMMERS, J., *and* RUNNSTRÖM, J. (1966). *Exptl Cell Res.* **43**, 444.
HÖRSTADIUS, S. *and* JOSEFSSON, L. (1972). *Acta Embryol. Morph. exp.* **14**, 7.
HÖRSTADIUS, S., JOSEFSSON, L., *and* RUNNSTRÖM, J. (1967). *Devl Biol.* **16**, 189.
HÖRSTADIUS, S., LORCH, J., *and* CHARGAFF, E. (1954). *Exptl Cell Res.* **6**, 440.
HÖRSTADIUS, S., LORCH, J., *and* DANIELLI, J. F. (1950). *Exptl Cell Res.* **1**, 188.
—— —— —— (1953). *Exptl Cell Res.* **4**, I 253, II 263.
HÖRSTADIUS, S. *and* STRÖMBERG, S. (1940). *W. Roux Arch. EntwMech. Org.* **140**, 409.
HÖRSTADIUS, S. *and* WOLSKY, A. (1936). *W. Roux Arch. EntwMech. Org.* **135**, 69.
HYNES, R. O. *and* GROSS, P. R. (1970). *Devl Biol.* **21**, 383.
IMMERS, J. *and* RUNNSTRÖM, J. (1965). *J. Embryol. exp. Morph.* **14**, 289.
JANSSENS, F. A. (1904). *Cellule.* **21**, 245.
JENKINSON, J. W. (1911*a*). *Arch. EntwMech. Org.* **32**, 269.
—— (1911*b*). *Arch. EntwMech. Org.* **32**, 699.
JOSEFSSON, L. *and* HÖRSTADIUS, S. (1969). *Devl Biol.* **20**, 481.
JUST, E. E. (1919). *Biol. Bull. mar. biol. Lab., Woods Hole,* **36**, 1.
KING, T. J. *and* BRIGGS, R. (1956). *Cold Spring Harb. Symp. quart. Biol.* **21**, 271.
KOEHLER, O. (1914). *Ber. naturf. Ges. Freiburg i. B.* **20**, 75.
—— (1916). *Z. indukt. Abstamm.- u. VererbLehre.* **15**, 1.
KÜHN, A. (1955). *Vorlesungen über Entwicklunsphysiologie.* Springer, Berlin.
LALLIER, R. (1955). *Archs Biol., Liège.* **65**, 75.
—— (1959*a*). *J. Embryol. exp. Morph.* **7**, 540.
—— (1959*b*). *Experientia.* **15**, 228.
—— (1962). *J. Embryol. exp. Morph.* **10**, 563.
—— (1964). *Adv. Morphogen.* **3**, 147.
—— (1966). *Ann. Biol.* 5, 313.
—— (1968). *Acta Embryol. Morph. exp.* **10**, 280.
—— (1969). *C. r. Séanc. Soc. Biol.* **163**, 2028.
LANDAUER, W. (1922). *Arch. EntwMech. Org.* **52**, 1.
LEHMANN, F. E. (1956). *Einführung in die physiologische Embryologie.* Verlag Birkhäuser, Basel.
LENIQUE, P. S., HÖRSTADIUS, S. *and* GUSTAFSON, T. (1953). *Exptl Cell Res.* **5**, 400.
LILLIE, F. (1912). *Science.* **36**, 527.

LILLIE, F. (1919). *Problems of fertilization.* University Chicago Press.

LINDAHL, P. E. (1932*a*). *W. Roux Arch. EntwMech. Org.* **126**, 373.

—— (1932*b*). *W. Roux Arch. EntwMech. Org.* **127**, 300.

—— (1932*c*). *W. Roux Arch. EntwMech. Org.* **127**, 323.

—— (1933). *W. Roux Arch. EntwMech. Org.* **128**, 61.

—— (1935). *Ark. Zool.* **B28**, no. 24.

—— (1936). *Acta zool., Stockh.* **17**, 179.

—— (1937). *Biol. Zbl.* **57**, 389.

—— (1941*a*). *Acta zool., Stockh.* **22**, 101.

—— (1941*b*). *Naturwissenschaften.* **29**, 673.

LINDAHL, P. E. and HOLTER, H. (1940). *C. r. Lab. Carlsberg, ser. chim.* **23**, 257.

LINDAHL, P. E. and LUNDIN, J. (1948). *Science,* **108**, 481.

LINDAHL, P. E. and NYBERG, E. (1955). *I.V.A. Stockh.* **26**, 309.

LINDBERG, O. (1943). *Ark. Kemi Miner. Geol.* **A16**, no. 15.

—— (1945). *Ark. Kemi Miner. Geol.* **B20**, no. 1.

—— (1946). *Ark. Kemi. Miner. Geol.* **A23**, no. 2.

LOEB, J. (1899). *Am. J. Physiol.* **3**, 135.

—— (1908). *Arch. EntwMech. Org.* **26**, 82.

—— (1909). *Die chemische Entwicklungserregung des thierischen Eies.* Springer, Berlin.

LÖNNING, S. (1967). *Årbok Univ. Bergen. Mat.-naturv. Ser.* **5**, 1.

LÖNNING, S. and HAGSTRÖM, B. (1971). *Protoplasma.* **73**, 303.

LÖNNING, S. and WENNERBERG, C. (1963). *Sarsia.* **11**, 25.

LORCH, J., DANIELLI, J. F., and HÖRSTADIUS, S. (1953). *Exptl Cell Res.* **4**, 253.

LYON, E. P. (1906*a*). *Am. J. Physiol.* **15**, 21.

—— (1906*b*). *Arch. EntwMech. Org.* **23**, 151.

MAAS, O. (1901). *S. Ber. Ges. Morph. Physiol. Münch.* **17**, 14.

—— (1905). *Z. wiss. Zool.* **82**, 601.

MACBRIDE, E. W. (1906). *Echinodermata. Cambridge natural history,* Vol. 1, p. 456.

—— (1914). *Q. Jl. microsc. Sci.* **59**, 471.

—— (1918). *Q. Jl. microsc. Sci.* **90**, 323.

MARKMAN, B. (1958). *Acta zool., Stockh.* **39**, 103.

—— (1962). *Exptl Cell Res.* **25**, 224.

—— (1963). *Ark. Zool. Ser.* 2. **16**, 207.

—— (1967). *Exptl Cell Res.* **46**, 1.

MARKMAN, B. and RUNNSTRÖM, J. (1963). *Exptl Cell Res.* **31**, 615.

—— —— (1970). *W. Roux Arch. EntwMech. Org.* **165**, 1.

MARX, W. (1929). *Zool. Anz.* **80**, 331.

MASTRANGELO, M. F. (1966). *J. exp. Zool.* **161**, 109.

MCCLENDON, J. F. (1909). *Am. J. Physiol.* **23**, 460.

MOAR, V. A., GURDON, J. B., LANE, C. D., and MARBAIX, G. (1971). *J. mol. Biol.* **61**, 93.

MONROY, A. (1965). *Chemistry and physiology of fertilization.* Holt, Rinehart, and Winston, New York.

MORGAN, T. H. (1893). *Anat. Anz.* **8**, 803.

—— (1894). *Anat. Anz.* **9**, 141.

—— (1895*a*). *Arch. EntwMech. Org.* **2**, 65.

—— (1895*b*). *Arch. EntwMech. Org.* **2**, 72.

—— (1895*c*). *Arch. EntwMech. Org.* **2**, 81.

—— (1895*d*). *Arch. EntwMech. Org.* **2**, 257.

—— (1895*e*). *Arch. EntwMech. Org.* **2**, 268.

—— (1895*f*). *J. Morph.* **10**, 419.

References

181

MORGAN, T. H. (1901). *Arch. EntwMech. Org.* **13**, 416.

—— (1903). *Arch. EntwMech. Org.* **16**, 117.

—— (1905). *J. exp. Zool.* **2**, 495.

—— (1934). *Embryology and Genetics.* Columbia Univ. Press.

MORGAN, T. H. and LYON, E. P. (1907). *Arch. EntwMech. Org.* **24**, 147.

MORGAN, T. H. and SPOONER, G. B. (1909). *Arch. EntwMech. Org.* **28**, 104.

MORTENSEN, T. (1920). *Papers. Dept. mar. biol. Carnegie Inst. Washington.* **16**, 80.

MOSER, F. (1939). *J. exp. Zool.* **80**, 423.

MOTOMURA, I. (1941). *Sci. Rep. Tohoku Univ., Ser.* 4, **16**, 561.

—— (1948). *Sci. Rep. Tohoku Univ., Ser.* 4, **18**, 117.

—— (1953). *Exptl Cell Res.* **5**, 187.

—— (1960). *Sci. Rep. Tohoku Univ., Ser.* 4, **26**, 367.

MÜLLER, J. (1846). *Arch. Anat. Physiol. wiss. Med.*, p. 101.

—— (1848). *Über die Larven und die Metamorphose der Ophiuren und Seeigel.* Berlin. Vorgetragen in Königl. Akad. Wiss. Berlin 1846.

—— (1849). *Über die Larven und die Metamorphose der Echinodermen II.* Akad. Wiss. Berlin 1848.

NÜMANN, W. (1933). *Z. indukt. Abstamm. - u. VererbLehre.* **65**, 447.

OHSHIMA, H. (1922). *Q. Jl. microsc. Sci.* **66**, 105.

OKAZAKI, K. (1960). *Embryologia.* **5**, 283.

—— (1965). *Exptl Cell Res.* **40**, 585.

—— (1971). In *Cells in early development.* Iwanami Shoten Publ. Tokyo, p. 186.

—— (1972). *Symp. Cell Biol.* (Japan) **22**, 163.

PAINTER, T. S. (1915). *J. exp. Zool.* **18**, 299.

PALMER, I. (1935). *Biol. Bull. mar. biol. Lab., Woods Hole,* **69**, 336.

—— (1937). *Physiol. Zool.* **10**, 352.

PEASE, D. C. (1939). *J. exp. Zool.* **80**, 225.

—— (1941). *J. exp. Zool.* **86**, 381.

—— (1942a). *J. exp. Zool.* **89**, 329.

—— (1942b). *J. exp. Zool.* **89**, 347.

PERRIER, R. (1889). *Nouv. Archs Mus. Hist. nat., Paris,* **10**.

PETERFI, T. (1924). *Abderhaldens Handb. biol. Arbeitsmethoden,* Vol. 5, 2.

PLATT, J. B. (1893). *Anat. Anz.* **8**, 506.

PLOUGH, H. (1927). *Biol. Bull. mar. biol. Lab., Woods Hole,* **52**, 373.

—— (1929). *W. Roux Arch. EntwMech. Org.* **115**, 380.

POPA, G. T. (1927). *Biol. Bull. mar. biol. Lab., Woods Hole,* **52**, 238.

RANZI, S. (1962). *Adv. Morphogen.* **2**, 211.

RAUBER, A. (1886). *Zool. Anz.* **9**, 166.

ROTHSCHILD, LORD (1956). *Fertilization.* Methuen, London.

ROTHSCHILD, LORD and SWANN, M. M. (1952). *J. exp. Biol.* **21**, 469.

ROUX, W. (1885). *Z. Biol.* **21**, 3.

—— (1888a). *Virchows Arch. path. Anat. Physiol.* **114**, 113 and 246.

—— (1888b). *Biol. Zbl.* **8**, 405.

RUNNSTRÖM, J. (1914). *Arch. EntwMech. Org.* **40**, 526.

—— (1915). *Arch. EntwMech. Org.* **41**, 1.

—— (1917). *Arch. EntwMech. Org.* **43**, 223.

—— (1918a). *Arch. EntwMech. Org.* **43**, 409.

—— (1918b). *Arch. EntwMech. Org.* **43**, 432.

—— (1920). *Arch. EntwMech. Org.* **46**, 459.

—— (1923). *Acta zool., Stockh.* **4**, 285.

—— (1925a). *W. Roux. Arch. Entw Mech. Org.* **105**, 63.

—— (1925b). *W. Roux. Arch. Entw Mech. Org.* **105**, 114.

RUNNSTRÖM, J. (1925c). *Ark. Zool.* **B17**, no. 10.
—— (1925d). *Ark. Zool.* **A18**, no. 4.
—— (1926). *Acta zool., Stockh.* **7**, 117.
—— (1928a). *W. Roux Arch. EntwMech. Org.* **113**, 556.
—— (1928b). *Acta zool., Stockh.* **9**, 365.
—— (1928c). *Protoplasma.* **4**, 388.
—— (1929). *W. Roux Arch. EntwMech. Org.* **117**, 123.
—— (1930). *W. Roux Arch. EntwMech. Org.* **121**, 714.
—— (1931). *W. Roux Arch. EntwMech. Org.* **124**, 273.
—— (1933). *Protoplasma.* **20**, 1.
—— (1959). *Ark. Zool., Ser.* 2, **12**, 245.
—— (1962). *Exptl Cell Res.* **27**, 485.
—— (1964). In *Acidi nucleici e loro funzione biologica.* Istituto Lombardo, Fondazione Baselli, Milano, p. 342.
—— (1966a). *Adv. Morphogen.* **5**, 222.
—— (1966b). *Archo. zool. ital.* **51**, 239.
—— (1967). *Exp. Biol. Med.* **1**, 52.
RUNNSTRÖM, J., HÖRSTADIUS, S., IMMERS, J., and FUDGE-MASTRANGELO (1964). *Revue suisse Zool.* **71**, 21.
RUNNSTRÖM, J. and KRISZAT, G. (1952a). *Exptl Cell Res.* **3**, 419.
—— —— (1952b). *Exptl Cell. Res.* **3**, 497.
RUNNSTRÖM, J. and MARKMAN, B. (1966). *Biol. Bull. mar. biol. Lab., Woods Hole* **130**, 402.
RUNNSTRÖM, J. and RUNNSTRÖM, S. (1920). *Bergens Mus. Årb.* 1918–1919. *Naturvid. nr.* **5**, 1.
RUSTAD, R. C. (1960). *Acta Embryol. Morph. exp.* **3**, 155.
SCARANO, E. (1969). *Annls. embryol. Morphogen., Suppl.* **1**, 51.
—— (1971). *Adv. Cytopharmacology.* **1**, 13.
SCHAXEL, J. (1914). *Zool. Jb. Abt. Anat. Ont.* **37**, 131.
SCHJEIDE, O. A. (1970). Nuclear-cytoplasmic transfers. In *Cell differentiation (ed. Schjeide and De Vellis.)* van Nostrand Reinhold Comp., New York, p. 169.
SCHLEIP, W. (1929). *Die Determination der Primitiventwicklung.* Akad. Verlagsgesellschaft. Leipzig.
SCHMIDT, H. (1904). *Verh. phys.-med. Ges. Würzb.* **36**, 297.
SEELIGER, O. (1892). *Zool. Jb. Anat. Ont.* **6**, 161.
—— (1894). *Arch. EntwMech. Org.* **1**, 203.
—— (1896). *Arch. EntwMech. Org.* **3**, 477.
SELENKA, E. (1878). *Zoologische Studien. I. Befruchtung des Eies von Toxopneustes variegatus.* Leipzig.
—— (1883). *Die Keimblätter der Echinodermen.* I:2. Wiesbaden.
SHEARER, C., DE MORGAN, W., and FUCHS, H. M. (1914). *Phil. Trans. R. Soc.* **B 204**, 255.
SINISCALCO, M. (1969). *Excerpta Med. Int. Congr. Series,* No. 204, 72.
SPEK, J. (1918). *Kolloidchem. Beih.* **9**, 259.
SPEMANN, H. (1906). *Verh. dt. zool. Ges.* p. 195.
—— (1936). *Experimentelle Beiträge zu einer Theorie der Entwicklung.* Julius Springer, Berlin.
SPIEGEL, M. and TYLER, A. (1966). *Science.* **151**, 1233.
STEINBRÜCK, H. (1902). *Arch. EntwMech. Org.* **14**, 1.
STERN, H. (1970). Cellular and molecular events associated with mitosis and meiosis. In *Cell differentiation (Ed. Schjeide and de Vellis).* New York, p. 141.
STEVENS, N. M. (1902). *Arch. EntwMech. Org.* **15**, 421.

SWANN, M. M. (1954). *Pubbl. Stn. zool., Napoli*, **25**, 198.

TAYLOR, C. V. and TENNENT, D. H. (1924). *Yb. Carnegie Inst. Wash.*, **23**, 201.

TERNI, T. (1914). *Mitt. zool. Stn. Neapel.* **22**, 59.

THEEL, H. (1892). *Nova Acta R. Soc. Scient. upsal., Ser. III*, **15**, (6) 1.

THOMSON, W. (1865). *Phil. Trans. R. Soc.* **155**, 513.

TYLER, A. (1944). *Anat. rec.* **89**, 573.

—— (1948). *Physiol. Rev.* **28**, 180.

—— (1949). *The collecting net.* **19**, 19.

TYLER, A. and TYLER, B. S. (1966). In *Physiology of Echinodermata* (*Ed. Boolootian*). John Wiley and Sons, New York.

VASSEUR, E. (1948). *Acta Chem. scand.* **2**, 900.

VERNON, H. M. (1900). *Arch. EntwMech. Org.* **9**, 464.

VOGT, W. (1925). *W. Roux Arch. EntwMech. Org.* **106**, 542.

VON BAER, K. E. (1828). *Ueber Entwicke lungsgeschichte der Thiere.* Erster Teil. Gebrüder Bornträger, Königsberg.

—— (1847). *Bull. physico-math. Acad. imp. Sci. St. Petersbourg.* **5**, 231.

VON UBISCH, L. (1925a). *Z. wiss. Zool.* **124**, 361.

—— (1925b). *Z. wiss. Zool.* **124**, 457.

—— (1925c). *Z. wiss. Zool.* **124**, 469.

—— (1925d). *Verh. phys.-med. Ges. Würzb.* **50**, 13.

—— (1929). *W. Roux Arch. EntwMech. Org.* **117**, 80.

—— (1931). *W. Roux Arch. EntwMech. Org.* **124**, 181.

—— (1932a). *W. Roux EntwMech. Org.* **126**, 19.

—— (1932b). *W. Roux Arch. EntwMech. Org.* **127**, 216.

—— (1933). *W. Roux Arch. EntwMech. Org.* **129**, 45.

—— (1934). *W. Roux Arch. EntwMech. Org.* **131**, 95.

—— (1936). *W. Roux Arch. EntwMech. Org.* **134**, 599.

—— (1937). *Z. wiss. Zool.* **149**, 402.

—— (1939). *Biol. Rev.* **14**, 88.

—— (1954). *Pubbl. Stn. zool., Napoli*, **25**, 246.

—— (1957). *Pubbl. Stn. zool., Napoli*, **30**, 279.

—— (1959). *Pubbl. Stn. zool., Napoli*, **31**, 159.

WARBURG, O. (1908). *Hoppe-Seyler's Z. physiol. Chem.* **75**, 1.

WEISMANN, A. (1892). *Das Keimplasma. Eine Theorie der Vererbung.* Jena.

WESTIN, M. (1969). *J. exp. Zool.* **171**, 297.

WHEELER, W. M. (1898). *Arch. Biol.* **15**, 1.

WILSON, E. B. (1892a). *Anat. Anz.* **7**, 732.

—— (1892b). *J. Morph.* **6**, 361.

—— (1893). *J. Morph.* **8**, 579.

—— (1896). *Arch. EntwMech. Org.* **3**, 19.

—— (1903). *Arch. EntwMech. Org.* **16**, 40.

—— (1904). *J. exp. Zool.* **1**, 1 and 197.

WILSON, E. B. and MATTHEWS, A. P. (1895). *J. Morph.* **10**, 319.

WOLPERT, L. and GUSTAFSON, T. (1961). *Exptl Cell Res.* **25**, 311.

ZEUTHEN, E. (1951). *Pubbl. Stn. zool., Napoli. Suppl.* **23**, p. 47.

ZIEGLER, H. E. (1898). *Arch. EntwMech. Org.* **6**, 249.

ZOJA, R. (1895). *Arch. EntwMech. Org.* **2**, 1.

Author Index

Subject Index

acron, 17, 19
activation, 12, 14
animal
  and vegetal
    gradients, 43, 44
    halves as physiological tools, 166–71
  attraction power, 64, 65
  tuft, 17, 42
  –vegetal axis, 10, 14
  /vegetal balance, 50, 52, 61, 62, 161, 166, 171
animalization, 45
antifertilizin, 14
apex, 17, 19
apical tuft, *see* animal tuft
artificial
  insemination, 10
  sea-water, 31
attraction zone, 23, 55, 58
autonomous differentiation, 7
autonomy of life processes, 6

bilareral
  asymmetry, 119–33, 159
  organization, 42, 53, 92, 98, 158

calcium-free sea-water, 6, 31
centrifugation, 81–4
chimeras, 152
chromosomes and heredity, 134–7
cleavage and determination, 39, 163–5
coelomic vesicles, 113–33
constriction experiments, 34, 47, 93, 98, 120
cortical granules, 13
cytochromotidase activity, 106, 168
cytoplasmic inheritance, 141–51, 155–7

determination, 1
developmental
  biology, 2
  physiology, 2, 5

differentiation, 1
dispermy, 135
double gradients, 44, 122, 158

ectodermization, 45
egg axis, 10
ejection, 72, 155, 172
endododermization, 45, 54
endogenous morphogenetically active substances, 65. 164, 168–71
entelechy, 6
entrance cone, 13
Entwicklungsmechanik, 5
equatorial eggs, 14, 46
external agents, 73, 107, 166–71

fertilization, 10, 12
  cone, *see* entrance cone
  membrane, 13, 28
fertilizin, 14

gastrulation, 19, 22
genic action, 137, 141, 171
giants, 103
glass needles, 5, 9, 29
gradient, 7
grey crescent, 8
growth, 2

harmonious equipotential system, 6
heterosperm merogones, 138, 145
homosperm merogones, 138, 145
hyaline layer, 13
hybrid viability, 142

induction, 49, 53, 55, 58, 67, 153, 155, 156
inductive substances, 161, 162
isolation methods, 29, 112, 114, 118, 119

jelly layer, 11, 14, 28

labelled cells, 111, 162, 168

Species Index